How I Conquered Cancer Naturally

How I Conquered Cancer

Naturally

Eydie Mae
with Chris Loeffler

AVERY PUBLISHING GROUP INC.
Garden City Park, New York

ISBN 0-89529-518-0

Printed in the United States of America

10 9 8 7 6 5 4 3 2 1

CONTENTS

CHAPTER FIVE

CHAPTER SIX

CHAPTER SEVEN

CHAPTER EIGHT

CHAPTER NINE

APPENDIX

Dedicated to
my husband, Arn
without whose love, encouragement, and help
none of this would have happened.

My thanks to my good friend, Chris Loeffler, for the long hours spent at her typewriter, listening to us, taking heaps of notes, researching the details, compiling them all, and writing my story.

Eydie Mae

FOREWORD

This is not a scientific treatise on how to cure cancer. Neither is it a love story per se. This is a true story, a warm and intimate love story (but not in the usual sense), a practical and down-to-earth account of a courageous woman's march against death, with a detailed explanation of how she gained victory over perhaps the most dreaded disease of our time.

It must be clearly understood at the outset that Eydie Mae Hunsberger is a recovered cancer patient. Neither she, nor the author Chris Loeffler, are physicians; neither one nor the other is qualified to practice medicine in any way; neither the publisher nor the distributor is recommending anything in the treatment of cancer. If the reader is favorably impressed by the facts and opinions presented in the following pages, and if the reader decides to seek out Eydie Mae's method for his or her own use, the reader must do so entirely on his own evaluation of those facts and opinions, and not as a result of any "recommendation" on the part of Eydie Mae Hunsberger or Chris Loeffler.

This book will possibly be scoffed at, ridiculed, read with unbelief, and in general be highly controversial. Nonetheless, it is true, and Eydie Mae is the living proof, and her doctors, family and friends can verify what she has said.

1

THE MEDICAL APPROACH TO CANCER OF THE BREAST
(MASTECTOMY A MUST)

DISCOVERY

We had gone to bed that evening back in February, 1973. Our verbal communication had just about slowed down to a halt, when a long silence had stolen in upon us after Arn answered my sleepy but curious question, "What are you doing?"

"I've found something that I don't like," mused Arn.

My husband had found a lump, about the size of a quarter in my right breast.

My story starts right there.

Our national holiday, honoring Washington's birthday, prevented me from seeing my doctor until Tuesday. We carried on our normal activities and daily chores without panic the next day, but for me, it was as if the day was heavy and overcast with low threatening clouds, when in reality the sun was shining brightly and the air was as clear as only a February day in Southern California can be.

Arn was reassuring, concerned but optimistic, refusing to really consider the possibility of cancer, chiding me for worrying, trying to say something to cheer me up, but I think a little disappointed in me because I was so down. There was no denying my dark mood.

The fear and the feeling of despair that raced through my mind and body for the next two days were an agonizing nightmare. Over and over in my mind I asked the question, "What if it is cancer?" The uncertainty of not knowing the answer to that question was almost unbearable, yet there was nothing to do but wait in dreadful suspense. I couldn't remember ever feeling this fearful and apprehensive about anything before. Round and round in my head the same thought kept repeating itself, each time my heart sinking a little bit lower, with depression beating a lower, deadlier beat each time, "It could be cancer!"

I was petrified.

"Is there any disease that a woman dreads more?" I pondered.

My first thoughts were of Arn, my husband, "Supposing it is cancer...if I had to have my breast removed, how would I look to him? Would he find me physically repulsive? Dear God! I couldn't take that. Arn is as much a part of me as my breast...you might as well take my heart out, too."

"Slow down, Eydie Mae, you are *not* going to panic," I deliberately reminded myself.

"What silly thoughts!" I scolded myself. "I know perfectly well that Arn's love is constant and strong. He would never turn aside in the face of calamity or trouble. Many times I've seen him face trouble on the job, sometimes with people, sometimes just circumstances. He's always loyal to his workers, fighting for them unabashed at glaring faults, always giving them the benefit of the doubt; troubling circumstances to him are just something to find a way to overcome...and he does."

My mind wandered back over our lives together. Coming from German Swiss and Dutch stock, Arn has a passion for hard work and is highly disciplined. It was part of his upbringing as a child to be taught that work is a virtue and in his home he was given wise, sturdy discipline, the kind he could never forget.

There may have been times, when feeling sorry for myself, that I wondered whether he loved his work more than me, but all I had to do was to remind myself of his background and I knew that his work was part of him, just as I was and the rest of the family.

I thought of the birth of our son, twenty-seven years ago. Because of complications, the doctor felt that he had to give me a Caesarean operation when I was only seven months pregnant. They gave me a spinal anesthesia, feeling that this would give our baby the best possible chance. Our son was delivered without any problems, but I was left paralyzed from the waist down, incapable of caring for myself. That was another nightmare. The incision wouldn't heal despite all the antibiotics they kept pumping into me, and infection set in. One long month I was in the hospital. The doctors did everything they could to help me, to no avail. Feeling had been restored to my legs, but I was incapable of controlling by body functions, and the incision was still wide open and ugly with infection. Arn took me home, and carried me all around the house. We dropped all medication. Gradually, with utmost patience, he massaged my legs and spine and held me as I struggled to learn to walk again. With his alternately carrying me and helping me to walk, the incision started to drain of its own accord getting rid of the toxins that had been unaffected by medication. Gradually the infection cleared, the gaping hole closed up, and once again I could control my body functions. His loving care had turned the tide for us then.

"No, I certainly shouldn't question Arn's possible reactions," I rallied.

Fear. Fear does stange things to one's mind.

My mind still would not let me be. I thought of my good friend, Betty who had died of cancer after having the best possible care—all the treatments the medical field had to offer—everything money could buy.

Betty had had to have a radical mastectomy

because of breast cancer. As a result of this radical surgery, extending up under her arm and down to her elbow, then down and across her rib cage, she had had to wear long sleeves all the time because of her swollen arm. Not many months after that it had spread to other vital organs. She had loved life and had so much for which to live! She had been doggedly determined to continue with their plans to travel Europe the following year. Yet in spite of all those various treatments, she had died before she had ever been able to get there. I grieved again for my friend.

Then there was my friend, Mary, whose mother had been cut up piece by piece, as she slowly died of cancer. Her husband had made sure that she had the finest doctor in New York City, and the most advanced treatment available in the best hospital. It didn't make any difference. Her cancer had started in the cervix. After her uterus had been taken out, the surgeon had cut out her bladder which meant tubes forever coming out of her sides, then they had removed her large intestine and had relocated her anus in her lower abdomen. The emotional trauma involved with all this was excruciating. Her last year and a half she merely existed. In spite of the best treatment modern medicine could offer, and massive medical costs, she died.

"What could be in store for me?" I climbed on the merry-go-round again.

I was devastated when I thought about the pain and the agony that walks hand in hand with that dread disease, cancer.

"I've got to stop thinking this way," I rebelled, "I've got a lot of living to do yet. I'm not ready to die. This isn't real!"

Then I crumbled, one little grandson we had, and another on the way, "I want to see my grandchildren grow up. Am I not even going to be able to hold that new little wee one in my arms? The kids may want to do something and I won't be here to tell them how to do it." How awful it would be not to be a part of their lives anymore. I fought with these thoughts, trying not to be so pessimistic.

My thoughts came back home. Arn and I had been working so hard for so long—fourteen hours a day—seven days a week—building towards a day when we would enjoy more leisure and have more time together. The future had looked good. I had been dreaming of the day when we would start pouring over maps, and fascinating books and travel brochures getting ready to see something more of this wonderful world in which we lived. So many things we had planned. Now, maybe I wasn't going to be a part of the future. I wouldn't be able to reap the rewards from our long hours of labor.

What about Arn's parents? They had just come through a long period of illness and I didn't want to alarm them. We've been very close over the years. If this was cancer, how would this shock affect their health?

I had not yet made peace with my maker.

I was so at war with myself.

I was scared.

"Remember, Eydie Mae, you are not going to panic," I steadied myself again.

The lump, that unattractive, chilling word, wasn't *that* big, and we *had* caught it early. We had found the lump on Sunday and I was going to see the doctor on Tuesday.

Maybe everything was going to be all right.

I SEE MY FAMILY DOCTOR

Four months previous I had had a complete physical checkup. I had gone through all those uncomfortable tests. As well as a pap smear, my breasts had been thoroughly checked—nothing had been detected. My doctor had pronounced me to be as healthy as anyone could be.

How many times had I read about how important it was to have regular checkups? On that Tuesday I was no longer convinced of the validity of that argument.

My visit shook my doctor up as well as me. He checked over my records with the utmost care, being concerned lest he had overlooked anything back in October. There just hadn't been any indication only four months ago.

By manipulating the lump, he was immediately suspicious because it was not smooth (which would have indicated the probability of it being nonmalignant, or just a benign cyst). My lump was irregular and had what he described as a cancerous feeling to it. He ordered a mammogram (an X-ray of the breast).

After the mammogram was taken Tuesday afternoon, we had to wait another long day for the analysis. Reaching out for some hope to come from some source, I tried to get an indication from the radiologist. "I'm sorry, but you'll have to see your doctor," was his reply.

The following day, the reading of the mammogram pointed towards cancer. This was not a positive identification as it still depends on human analysis, but things were really beginning to look black.

My doctor recommended that I see a specialist in the field of cancer, and made an appointment for me to see a highly reputable surgeon.

I felt kind of numb, almost detached as if my doctor was talking to someone else. I didn't want to accept what he was telling me. I left his office in a daze, not remembering a thing that I said to him.

Then the impact suddenly reached me and I furiously wanted to strike back! If there had been a set of dishes within reach, I would have smashed them all against my doctor's adobe wall. Tears of rage engulfed me, as I ran to the car.

This couldn't be happening to me.

THE SPECIALIST

Up until this time, Arn had not allowed himself to believe that the lump could be cancerous. Anybody else, but just not his wife. After the reading of the mammogram, however, he became more than just concerned and decided to accompany me to see the cancer specialist.

Thank God Arn went with me to see the specialist, as I know I wasn't thinking too clearly and I needed his support for what was in store for me.

The surgeon's examination and diagnosis verified the opinion of our family doctor, and my stomach began to tie in knots.

He explained the next step—biopsy—or the need for a laboratory examination under a microscope of the lump to determine without a shadow of a doubt that it was or was not malignant.

According to him, it is regular medical procedure for the surgeon to open the breast, remove the tumor or cyst, then send it to the lab to be examined immediately. The patient is held under anesthesia on the operating table. If the tissue is benign, the surgeon would finish sewing up the biopsy incision and it would be all over. If the tissue is malignant, then the surgeon would perform a radical mastectomy.

A radical mastectomy is where the surgeon removes the breast and eighty percent of the lymph glands that are under the arm, almost to the elbow of the arm and down the side. Sometimes the underlying muscles around the rib cage are removed. The arm often remains swollen about twenty-five percent larger than normal and about twenty-five percent of the strength and mobility of the arm is lost. The arm doesn't swing as far and cannot be used to lift things. And of course, it would produce a most obvious cosmetic deformity which would be traumatic even when a person leads a well-balanced life and understands that vanity is an unworthy virtue.

Since we talked with this surgeon, I have read about a woman, a close friend of Shirley Temple Black's, who upon going into the hospital for a biopsy, had, it seemed, signed papers without fully comprehending the medical terminology, giving the surgical team advance permission to do whatever was judged best, depending on the pathological analysis of the lump. She had awakened from the operation without a breast, when she honestly had expected only a biopsy.

After talking it over, both Arn and I felt that a radical mastectomy was an extreme answer for my case and Arn began to question the doctor, "We caught this early, why not just take out the lump?"

The specialist's reaction to this suggestion was made without hesitation, "Impossible." He insisted that medically speaking, the only thing that was indicated in my case was a radical mastectomy. He would not even consider a lumpectomy (the removal of the lump only). Emphatically he made the point that the medical profession had been doing these things for fifty-five years and that they most certainly knew what they were doing.

Arn's ire was raised then and he suggested that if the doctors had been doing this for fifty-five years, they should have found a better solution by now. He started questioning their methods and their logic. The conversation became rather heated at this point, and the doctor was rather contemptuous of Arn's prodding. I guess no one usually questioned this good doctor's opinion.

Slowly, our specialist gained control of his anger and did admit that some modern doctors had started doing a simple mastectomy. They just removed the breast itself. They did not take out the muscles or the lymph glands as in a radical mastectomy. However, he remained adamant to the fact that he had had lots of experience and he would not even recommend a simple mastectomy, let alone a lumpectomy.

Then he really leveled with us and told us that surgery probably would not stop with a radical mastectomy as there was no guaranteed way to stop the cancer from spreading. All we could do was hope. If the disease progressed, they would take out my ovaries, then my adrenal glands, and then my pituitary gland along with giving me radiation, all to keep me alive and give me more time.

By the time he was finished with that list, I had a horrible sinking feeling in the pit of my stomach, and was overwhelmed with uncertainty and fear. All I wanted to do right then was get out of there and escape what I was hearing. This was serious, far more serious than I had allowed myself to think and I felt that I couldn't begin to make an intelligent decision under the duress of the moment.

Without any conviction whatsoever, I agreed with Arn that I still preferred that just the lump be taken out, but that I really didn't *know* which way to go. In my mind I seriously questioned whether we should consult another doctor.

The surgeon continued, "There is no known cure for cancer, we can't claim a cure. The best I can tell you is that you have an eighty percent chance to live one year, and a maximum life expectancy of five years."

Arn exclaimed, "That's not good enough! I've been hearing things on television, things that have been coming from the medical profession, not quackery. I've seen the Cancer Society literature that indicates that cancer is easily curable if caught in the early stages." (Copy from one such American Cancer Society ad reads: Once a year, even if you're feeling terrific, see your doctor for a checkup. A checkup can detect cancer before any signs or symptoms appear. *And early enough for your doctor to do something about it.* Don't be afraid. *Cancer is one of the most curable of the major diseases in the U.S. today.* But it *must* be caught early.)

The doctor came back with, "No, you'll never see anything that says there is a cure for cancer. I have to give you the straight statistics. We think that this is the best way to do it, and we just feel that we shouldn't be kidding people at this stage."

Looking back on it, we feel we were fortunate that he leveled with us and did not give us any false hope, or we probably would have chosen to go the conventional way.

Before we left, refusing to believe that we might not take his authoritative advice, the surgeon insisted on calling the hospital and setting me up in three days for the operation, a radical mastectomy. We parted with his statement ringing in our ears, "I want you in the hospital in three days!"

2 | THREE LONG DAYS

THE NEXT STEP

Long after we left the doctor's office, Arn was still arguing with him. "There must be something else! In my business, the customer has every right to question me and he does. And sometimes we've gotten new ideas from just such encounters. The customer is king in my business. That surgeon was like an ant on an apple who thought the whole world was red, just because people never question his decision or methods. There must be something else."

My mind wasn't operating very efficiently. I couldn't get any further than thinking about the radical mastectomy. Three days until the operation —oh how I didn't want that operation. Was there really any alternative?

After much more discussion, Arn and I decided to read everything we could find about breast cancer. We called all over the country seeking help in getting references and in those next three long days we read approximately twenty books.

There was one very helpful group called "Cancer Victims and Friends." This is *not* a part of the well-known American Cancer Society which we hear so much about. They have a bookstore in Solana Beach, California. We found reams of information there, almost a whole shelf of books in the local library and many books in health food stores. We literally read everything we could get our hands on.

In book after book, the reality and the seriousness of the subject hit us full in the face. Round and round in our heads we asked, "How could the doctor be so set in his ways when there seemed to be so many failures? How many cures have there been? Does anyone even have their cancer under control? How could other people be so sure their ways should be tried? We surely weren't turning up any great numbers of successes.

Hundreds of books to choose from. How were we to pick them out?

Ice cream, vanilla and chocolate, but what when there are thirty-one flavors? (With the printing of this book, you now have the 32nd flavor).

We had to find that elusive bit of knowledge somewhere that would put us on the right track to a better way. Would we find it in print? Did it even exist?

WE TELL THE FAMILY

I didn't want to tell the family, let alone my

friends. I found that I couldn't really say what was on my mind. I didn't want to have to explain what I was going through. My own personal world was upside down.

I had been orphaned at an early age, so I didn't have to break the news to *my* parents, but can you keep your misery from those you love? There was no way out. As much as we didn't want to, we had to break the news to our children and to Arn's parents, and so we did.

Right away they wanted to know when and where the operation was going to be. When I told them we were thinking of the possibility of not having the operation, I could feel their concern and confusion and their feeling of helplessness and of unbelief. "What other way is there to go? What in the world are you thinking of doing? Why?" they queried, while trying to understand. They put some very real pressures on us that built up and grew on us day by day.

After Arn's parents had thought about it for some time, his mother called back and confided, "I've done all my crying. You're old enough to make your own decisions. Now tell me all about it."

Our daughter is married and living in another state, so she wasn't close enough to register too much static.

Our son, Bob didn't let us off quite so easily. He is an intelligent, levelheaded engineer, who graduated top student at San Diego State College in Engineering. We regard him very highly.

Bob didn't normally challenge Arn's reasoning. He respects his father's intelligence and is well acquainted with Arn's method of attacking problems. Arn was used to steam rollering a problem through to a good answer or very often to a *better* way. Normally, our son would get with the project and become as enthused as Arn, but this time he failed to join the momentum and get on the bandwagon. He saw Arn attacking this problem like any other problem, and he felt that this was more serious than just another problem.

Arn told me that our son came to him and told him that he thought this operation was not Arn's decision to make, but his mother's. Bob felt that Arn had been more or less pulling the strings, and he didn't think Arn was seeing it from every angle. In anguish, he asked the question, "What if you make a mistake? If you weren't trying to do it your way, mother could possibly have five years. What if the doctors are right and there is no viable alternative? You can't back up and start over as we have done so many times with mechanical problems."

After considerable thought, Arn decided our son was right, it really was my decision, and he let me know that no matter what I decided, he was with me.

MY DECISION

What *did* I want to do? And Arn? Was a wife's

decision ever fully her own? How was I to decide?

The first thing I decided to do was to tell my close friends, and share my dilemma.

La Verne wept and cried out, "You little twerp, I thought it would be me." She had always had a fear of cancer. She understood my thinking about not wanting the radical mastectomy, but she thought that if it were she, she would follow the doctor's advice.

Dee (registered nurse) knew of a few successes and without hesitation said that if it were her decision, she would go the conventional way, but she didn't pressure me.

The phone started ringing, "We just heard and we are so sorry, when is the operation?" It seemed like the phone never stopped ringing after that. People are great. So many wanted to help. Not one of my friends thought there was any alternative to the medical diagnosis and answer.

I got a good case of feeling sorry for myself, thinking maybe Arn and I were being unrealistic, shooting for a star on some far off horizon that would never come into clear focus. Confusion and frustration were reigning supreme within me. Then I realized that what I really wanted was someone else to agree with me that there could be another answer—some other moral support. Then I got mad.

I got mad at the cancer.

I got mad at the pressures of the world.

I got mad at myself for wanting to lean on

friends. I suddenly saw clearly that in man's hour of need, he really stands alone, but I also saw that in *my* hour of need Arn stood with me and I have never appreciated my husband more than in that moment of "knowing" what this mystical union really is between husband and wife that makes them "one." I suddenly knew that I could have the radical mastectomy, and although my thinking would be different than Arn's if I decided that way, he would accept me and my thinking, stand by me, support me, and continue to love me—and I was filled with thankfulness.

I started the mental fight to win.

Our specialist had told me that they could retard cancer by surgery, but couldn't cure it. He had outlined my destiny. To be taken apart, piece by piece, ending in certain death wasn't much to look forward to, nor did I want to burn up from radiation. I'd seen it all happen too often. Whether I had months, or a year or five years, I decided I wanted to live the rest of my life as a whole person rather than under the threat of continuous surgery and misery.

It was the hardest decision I ever had to make. I didn't know whether I was right, but from the depths of my being I felt that I wanted to search out another way. If there was one to be found.

I saw our government pouring millions of dollars into research grants to find a cure for cancer. With all that money working for me, I figured they just might find a cure within the next year. If I could stretch my luck that long, maybe I could buy a pill to cure cancer over the drugstore counter by this time next year. That was one of my biggest hopes.

I decided to just have the lump removed. Our family doctor was incredulous with surprise and tried to argue us out of it. When he finally became convinced that he could not sway us, he told Arn that he (Arn) would have to call the surgeon and cancel the operation.

Arn called my surgeon and when he cancelled the radical mastectomy, Arn took a tongue lashing like he had never taken before or since. Irritated to the point of disgust, the surgeon reprimanded Arn saying there should be laws against people like him. It was a hard thing to withstand the verbal castigation that came from this medical authority. No way would he perform the lumpectomy. Again he chastised Arn, telling him that he could hold himself directly responsible for my ensuing death. Their conversation ended with, "You're telling me that I should cancel the operation? OK, that's it then—you're going to *kill* that woman!"

IMMUNOTHERAPY

Not too long after making this decision, a new and still experimental treatment was brought to our attention, a treatment called immunotherapy which uses a biochemical strategy designed to trick the body's own natural defenses into fighting cancer.

An article in Time Magazine described immunotherapy as, "the rapidly expanding science of self-immunology—the study of the body's natural defenses against disease. That science is one of the most promising weapons yet developed by doctors in their long fight against cancer, which this year alone will afflict an estimated 650,000 Americans and kill more than 350,000. The older techniques— surgery, radiation and chemotherapy (drug treatments)—have been used successfully in bringing some cancers under control. But surgery usually results in unsightly and handicapping mutilation, radiation can destroy healthy as well as cancerous tissue, and chemotherapy produces unpleasant and dangerous side effects. Immunotherapy, which so far seems to have none of these disadvantages, could thus prove to be the ideal approach." [1]

In the same article, Dr. Lloyd Old, vice-president and associate director of the Sloan-Kettering Institute for Cancer Research, said, "Let's think of control of cancer rather than cure. Cancer is not a killing disease; what kills is progressive cancer. What we're trying to do is not eliminate cancer but establish an equilibrium between cancer and its hosts."

The article further stated that "doctors cannot

make immunotherapy work for all patients. They have no sure way of knowing who will respond until they begin treatment."

Arn and I talked this over and thought that maybe this was what we were searching for and decided to find out if there was some way to get me into this kind of a research program. More phone calls and research succeeded in searching out a doctor who was using this immunology approach in treating cancer patients. This doctor believes that malignant cancer is an infection that is caused by a microbial agent that lies dormant in most of us until our natural immunological defenses are weakened by illness, aging, a poor genetic immunological system, poor diet, or some trauma in our lives at which time these microbial agents can form an army and take over. If this premise is true, (and I believe it is) then surgery, radiation, and chemicals would not eradicate a continuing infectious process, but vaccine obtained from the patient's own tissues and body fluids could possibly treat the underlying infection and raise the general immunity.

The doctor agreed to take me into his program of testing and treating. Arn and I had great hopes that it would work for me.

After my past history was all recorded, many tests were made, and as I recall, the treatment proceeded as follows:

    1. In the beginning a urine culture was made twice a week and the organisms were isolat-

ed and used to prepare an autogenous vaccine.

2. Dark field and bright field microscopic examinations of my blood were done on every visit.
3. Antibiotic Sensitivity Tests were made.
4. All poultry products including eggs (even in baking) were eliminated from my diet.
5. All sugars were eliminated since many of these organisms live in the intestinal tract and multiply in great numbers during fermentation of sugars and starches.
6. White flour was forbidden since it is lacking in good nutritive elements.
7. No smoking was allowed.
8. No alcohol was permitted because the detoxification of alcohol puts a tremendous strain on the liver.
9. I was given the anti-tuberculosis vaccine, BCG, (Bacillus Calmette Guerin) in an attempt to activate all the fighting forces within my body to get my own immunization working.
10. Gamma globulin was also administered.
11. Proper nutrition and vitamin therapy to further support the body's defense mechanism was another important part of the treatment.
12. All chemicals, cleaning solutions, solvents such as paint removers and insect sprays were to be avoided, as all toxic materials are

detoxified in the liver and a liver already trying to cope with disease cannot sustain further stress.

The doctor suggested that I see a surgeon and have a simple mastectomy or at the very least a lumpectomy so that my system would not have as much cancer to overcome. What a battle we had to find a doctor who would perform a simple lumpectomy on me!

3 | THE UNCONVENTIONAL WAY

THE LUMPECTOMY

Our family doctor adamantly refused to do a lumpectomy or to help me get one, all the time insisting that we would be unable to get another doctor to do it either. For a time it appeared that he was right. We contacted a number of other doctors, but the very least they would consider doing was to perform a simple mastectomy.

In this country, Dr. George Crile, Jr. from Cleveland, Ohio, pioneered the lumpectomy operation. We had read some books by him and admired his courage, feeling that he must be a strong individual, not to follow the generally accepted practice.

In April of 1965, Dr. Crile published a scientific paper in the American Journal of Surgery, Vol. 109 on the "Treatment of Breast Cancer by Local Excision." One of the reports mentioned in his article is as follows:

"In 1943 Adair reported a large series of cases in which most of the patients had been treated by radical mastectomy with or without radiation, but a few had been treated by simple mastectomy or local excision of the tumors with or without radiation. There is a slight discrepancy between the figures mentioned by Adair in the text and those tabulated; however, in both the tables and the text there is a higher rate of survival in patients treated by simple operations than by radical procedures." (Tables I, II, III) [1]

TABLE I

FIVE YEAR SURVIVAL AFTER SURGERY ONLY

No. of Cases	Type of Operations	Survivors [percent]
172	Radical mastectomy	63
14	Simple mastectomy	72
8	Local excision	88

TABLE II

FIVE YEAR SURVIVAL AFTER PREOPERATIVE RADIATION AND SURGERY

No. of Cases	Type of Operations	Survivors [percent]
582	Radical mastectomy	49
30	Simple mastectomy	54
31	Local excisions	58

TABLE III

FIVE YEAR SURVIVAL AFTER SURGERY AND
POSTOPERATIVE RADIATION

No. of cases	Type of Operations	Survivors [percent]
277	Radical mastectomy	54
30	Simple mastectomy	73
31	Local excisions	71

Another quote mentioned in his report is: "Keynes, an early proponent of simple operations, quoted Murley as saying, 'Since it is clearly difficult to effect any appreciable addition to the quantity of life, more attention should be paid to the quality of life.' In this context there are situations in which surgeons should not hesitate to treat cancer of the breast by simple excision. Both our experiences and the experience of others who have treated patients in this way indicate that, provided the primary tumor is completely removed, the extent of the operation has little or no effect on the patient's chances of survival."

The summary of his article is as follows:

"1. The five year survival rate of a group of twenty patients with cancer of the breast treated by local excision of the tumors was as high (65 percent) as that of a much larger group treated by complete mastectomy with or without axillary dissection or radiation. The patients were selected for local excision because of the peripheral location of their tumors. The lesions did not differ significantly in size, stage, or histology from the series with which they were compared.

2. There are several series of cases reported in the literature in which local excisions of breast lesions with or without radiation have yielded as high or higher proportions of five year survivals as did more radical operations.

3. It is not recommended that breast tumors be treated routinely, or even commonly by local excision: however, in special situations when there are important emotional or professional factors to consider, it is possible to select peripherally located lesions that can be excised locally with confidence that the rate of survival will be as high as is commonly seen after radical operations." [2]

We decided to telephone Dr. Crile, and we managed to get through and talked with him at length. According to him, he was accepting about thirty percent of the women who came to him for a lumpectomy, depending upon the condition of the lump.

My lump was the size of a quarter and about one quarter of an inch thick, located in the tissue underneath the nipple, but not attached to it. We figured it was in a pretty good spot for a lumpectomy. He couldn't promise anything, but he would see us if we would fly back to Cleveland.

At home, the phone was still ringing off the hook. Ninety-nine percent of our world was not agreeing with us. This was heartrending—really discouraging.

I had heard of the soldier who was marching on his left foot when everyone else in the company was marching on their right, yet he insisted that they were out of step and that he was right. God help us if this was the case with us.

We made our appointment with Dr. Crile, made our hotel reservations and bought our plane tickets. We had one last possibility to cover before we went to Cleveland.

We had heard of a doctor in town whose father had recently died of cancer of the neck. His was another case where he had watched the surgeon operate time after time, taking his father apart piece by piece, only to see him die a miserable death.

In hopes that he would be in sympathy with our plight, we decided to make one last stand and visit him, seeking a local doctor to do the lumpectomy.

We left in plenty of time to get to the airport in case our visit with the doctor was unsuccessful.

Evidently this was our day. After an enlightening discussion with this doctor, he agreed with us, feeling that it was possible in this early stage that we might have success with a simple lumpectomy in conjunction with the immunology program. He called a surgeon associate and made arrangements for the lumpectomy to be done locally.

Our first battle had been won by our stubborn persistence.

The hospital was able to make room for me right away, and I was extremely careful when I signed the papers in the hospital that I was agreeing only to the removal of the lump, nothing else. I strongly believed that as far as was humanly possible, what happened to me should be my own decision. I didn't want any surprises waiting for me when I came out from under the anesthesia.

By now, my sense of dread had been somewhat dissipated and my hopes were high that we had caught this in time. Hope is a strong ally. Right up to the laboratory report, Arn was sure that the lump was benign.

The lumpectomy was performed and the laboratory report came back bringing all of our worst fears to a head. The lump was malignant. Dread seized a new hold on my heart. Had we caught it in time? Only time was going to tell the rest of my story. I've never been one to wish away my life, but I wished with all my heart that I could look into the future and see what was in store for me. Had I made the right choice?

SHORT-TERM PROGRESS

Temporary relief came with the lumpectomy operation performed. The surgeon felt that he had been able to remove all the cancerous tissue and he had seen no tentacles. The skill with which he had performed the operation had left me with an almost undetectable amount of deformation or scarring. I was beginning to feel good about it all.

Arn and I continued our reading and research, only this time it wasn't quite so frantic. Laughter, fun and relaxation returned for a short time besides a normal work schedule.

My immunology program kept me busy. There were frequent visits for consultation, treatment and testing. Then there was a long list of things to be taken regularly—the autogenous vaccine, the BCG, gamma globulin, antibiotics, vitamins and food supplements.

Unfortunately, my use of the antibiotics turned out to be a harrowing experience. I was allergic to them all. It wasn't too long after we started with them that I was convinced that the antibiotics were going to do me in long before the cancer would have a fighting chance to catch up with me again.

I had broken out with the most awful case of hives. Big sections of my skin, some of them six inches in diameter and some ten inches in diameter had raised just like giant water blisters all over my body. OH HOW I ITCHED—and I didn't dare scratch them. What agonizing torment! I couldn't lie down. I couldn't sleep. I had such a deep intense burning itch that I had to walk the floor for hours utterly exhausted with no way to get relief.

It only took hours for me to react to the antibiotics, but it took three or four days each time to overcome the allergic reactions by taking other drugs to counteract these horrible side effects.

After the giant blisters, another antibiotic had been tried and I had broken out in little yellow blisters. Another one that was normally used to clear up bladder infections, gave me a bladder problem.

We finally decided that it just didn't seem worthwhile for me to continue in this particular area of the immunology program and so I abandoned the antibiotics, but continued with the rest.

Large doses of vitamins and minerals had been prescribed by the doctor to further support my defense mechanism. All in all, one day at lunch I counted thirty pills to be taken. It was difficult for me to adjust my thinking to the idea that these pills were food given to supplement my diet. The reality of the numbers of the pills was too much before me. After all those pills, who needed lunch?

Months went by: I was beginning to feel like a pin cushion from all the needles of my autogenous vaccine, BCG's and gamma globulin. Then came a crushing blow. My malignancy reared its ugly head again, more lumps. This time there were four under my right arm in the lymph glands and two located right under the surgeon's incision line.

How does one regroup, figure new tactics, and march again in opposition to such a relentless enemy?

DEEP DEPRESSION

Our high hopes for a positive response to the immunology program came tumbling down to the ground. Every indication now seemed to point toward the fact that immunology hadn't worked for me. Others we have heard and read about, yes, but my particular kind of carcinoma breast cancer turned out to be a tough case. The bottom dropped out of my world again.

We had continued searching out what was happening in the cancer field. We had heard of people getting favorable results from using Amegdalyn (the highly controversial food supplement, Laetrile). I tried this. We were unable to obtain Amegdalyn manufactured in the United States so we purchased some of European origin. After a period of time, it became evident that my response to this treatment was not favorable either, so we stopped this. (Some time later we discovered that in order for Amegdalyn to be helpful, it cannot be over-refined. There is every possibility that this is the reason why I didn't have success with it.)

Finding that "better way" seemed to be getting more elusive all the time. It appeared as though nothing we had tried so far had succeeded in even starting a reversal in my particular case.

Pain had now become a daily part of my living.

Continued testing in the immunology program showed my urine colony count (just one of the tests used to follow the progress of the disease) was increasing, now up to three hundred.

Everything was pointing towards a radical mastectomy again. Only this time the ovaries were supposed to go at the same time because they were getting hard and swollen.

"Should I let them take me apart? Should I die with tubes sticking in and out of me?" I agonized over this one.

My hair had grown coarse.

My appetite was gone.

A terrible weakness like none I had ever experienced before was devastating me. Sleep no longer refreshed me. I went to bed tired and awakened more tired.

I had so vigorously defended my right to do with my body exactly what I had decided was best. I had been so sure I didn't want to be cut up in pieces. Now doubts haunted me. Had I made the right choice? Had I decided the best way to go?

Then I recalled reading a story in one of the books we had researched, about a woman, a patient who had sought out a new doctor after having had a radical mastectomy, both ovaries removed, cobalt treatments, more lumps, more X-ray treatment, more lumps on her neck, more radiation, male hormones, bone destruction, liver impairment, chemotherapy, more hormone treatment, and then the removal of her adrenal glands.

The doctor had described with compassion the examination of this patient:

"We removed the covering sheet from her body. Experienced physicians that we are, we could only look at her with anguish and a sense of self-guilt that our profession had not rescued her from this dread disease but had mutilated her beyond recognition. The dark-rimmed, beautiful eyes; the hairy, coarse, yellow face; the angry, furrowed, deep red of the rhinoceros skin of her neck and chest; the nodules and ulcerations overlying the old mastectomy scar; the swollen abdomen with the wide transverse scars; the scars across her back; the thin, swollen legs; the tremendously distorted right arm; the bent and shrunken body—was this once a lovely bride, a loving mother, a tender wife, a friend, a good neighbor, a woman concerned for her community, her country, her world? A spiritual being clothed in flesh?

"As I placed my arm across her shoulders in an involuntary gesture of compassion, she whispered, 'They said it would be better this time but I am no better; I am worse. There is no more help. I won't let my husband see me anymore nor sleep in the same room. I must spare him this agony. How much longer can I keep up? Doctor, shall I kill myself?"[3]

Remembering this story, I knew that I had made the right decision, it was just so hard to think straight under the stress of the moment.

Deep depression brought utter confusion again. My thoughts tumbled over one another going round and round again in my head making me hate myself. Discouragement, disillusionment, and depression were having a heyday inside my mind:

"Arn is a busy executive, the president of a multi-million dollar business. He had guests to entertain. He needs me. I want to be by his side. We still have so many things we want to do together.

"If I could just stretch it out, they could discover that medical cure! How could they spend so much money and not find a cure? I'm dying, doesn't anybody care?

"I'm so weak.

"I feel so ugly.

"I feel so helpless.

"I feel so defeated.

"Why don't I just fly away and die?

"...............I don't want to die."

4 | A NEW DIRECTION

A REMARKABLE HAPPENING

It was a very somber dinner, unlike our sur-roundings. Arn and I were eating at the Gate-keeper Restaurant in La Jolla, California, a charming place overlooking the residences that lead down the hill to the beautiful Pacific Ocean. Specializing in salads, raw foods, and having hanging plants in a garden cottage like atmosphere, the Gatekeeper is well-known as a natural food restaurant, and worthy of its good reputation.

We were reviewing our problem.

We were read and researched to death.

It seemed like there were only two possibilities left—a nutritionist in Texas, or a radical mastec-tomy and ovary removal, the way of the surgeon's knife.

While we were going over our alternatives, we started talking about a woman, Wynn Davis, who lived in town. She supposedly knew a lot of people with cancer. She would know those who were having failures but also those who were having successes. Perhaps we could find her.

I was terribly tired, to the point of exhaustion.

I silently mused over the idea that here was one last meal where I could still get out. I could still get around. I wondered how long I could keep it up.

Then a miracle.

A lovely couple sitting at the table next to us got up and came over to our table. "I would like to introduce myself, I think I heard my name mentioned. I am Wynn Davis," the woman said. The gentleman with her was Bill Turner.

This remarkable and timely meeting shot a spark of hope into my heart.

We made arrangements to meet with her after she had eaten.

We asked her about herself and what had led her into the cancer fight. She told us about her son who had died of cancer at the age of twenty-one. She had seen him die an agonizing death and she was convinced that there must be another way. This was what created such determination in her to help others with cancer.

Wynn is everything that we had heard, a truly wonderful person. She was enthusiastic with an intellectual vigor and an unquenchable desire to serve others. She was immediately genuinely concerned about me and desirous of doing anything that she could to help us. We talked for a long time that first evening that we met.

We must have been talking for at least thirty

minutes when Arn turned to her and asked, "What if you had cancer? You've seen so many cases. Would you submit to surgery? Does it really matter what we do? Or is it really hopeless no matter what we do? If you were in our position and wanted to do the thing that you thought was the very best, what would you do?"

She was silent in her thoughts for awhile, then turned and discussed a few alternatives with her friend, Bill Turner. They carried on a long dialogue, first about one treatment and then another. They seemed to come by the decision with difficulty. Finally Bill suggested Ann Wigmore. In moments they had both agreed—then asked us, "Have you thought of Ann Wigmore?"

We had read about Ann Wigmore and the Hippocrates Health Institute, but had just not considered her "wheatgrass" and her theories on how to regenerate the human body as a likely alternative to cancer.

Bill said, "If it was me, I would go to Boston and stay with Ann Wigmore and do exactly what she says." Wynn echoed her agreement with him.

We pondered over this unexpected turn of events. As we were hashing over the reasons for their suggestion, my thoughts wandered back to a spot that had left its mark on my memory.

There is a small but lovely park area directly in front of the main railroad station in downtown Los Angeles. My husband and I had lingered there one day when we had had some time to spare before taking a train. On a very attractive sundial in this park, the following words are inscribed:

"Have the vision to see, the faith to believe, and the courage to do." I had memorized these words years ago. Perhaps they held some wisdom that could be applied to my circumstances that evening. We examined their suggestion from every angle we could. I certainly didn't like any of my other alternatives.

We finally decided that with the experience that these two people had had in trying to help others with cancer, there was every chance they had been inspired with the vision to see a better way for us. We stepped out in faith, believing this to be true, and found the courage to decide to "go to Boston, and stay with Ann Wigmore and do exactly what she said to do."

ANN WIGMORE AND THE MANSION

We decided to delay telling our doctor about our decision to go to Boston. In a matter of days, we made all the arrangements. Arn called Ann Wigmore and we were fortunate enough to have a reservation open up for the following week. Arn took two weeks off from the office and flew back with me to Boston. He wasn't about to send me off to some unknown institution without his checking it out personally. Knowing what I do now about Ann Wigmore's program, I don't think I could have gone through it alone and been successful. My energy was at such a low ebb, and my personal discomfort was so great by this time that I really needed the tender loving care and encouragement that Arn provided. Inside me, there was nothing calm, cool and collected. I was scared and I was desperate. This was the state of my mind when we arrived in Boston.

We had been told that Hippocrates Health Institute was located in an old mansion, so our imaginations had dreamed up an estate with grounds and so forth. Imagine our surprise when our cab pulled up in front of a five-story brownstone building very similar to the brownstones in New York City in an older part of town, very close to the business section.

We stood there wondering about it all, hoping this wasn't a wild goose chase.

Upon entering, it was nothing like a hospital, or a clinic, or a school, or anything other than a large old home with a quiet library like atmosphere.

There was a fellow sitting at the desk reading a book. There wasn't anybody running around in white coats and masks or nurses in white stockings pushing oxygen tanks or other medical equipment around; nor long forms to fill out with medical history or health records or health insurance. In fact, no one seemed to be the least bit concerned about the state of our health.

Ann Wigmore came down from her quarters on the fifth floor to greet us. Again, no interview, no questions about our complaints, just congenial concern that we be placed in the right room, that we be made comfortable, that we be made aware of the meal schedule (no menus to choose from) rather than the thing that was heavy on our minds, our serious problem with cancer.

I found out later why she did not show the concern I was looking for; she felt that I would get better if I stayed and really followed through with her program. So she was more concerned with making us comfortable.

We were assigned a room on the fourth floor. Our luggage went up in the elevator. We walked up. The elevator was very small, and it is one of Ann Wigmore's rules that everyone always walks.

Knowing how we Americans have grown so used to using mechanical means for getting around, she figured that even if we never came to exercise class, she could indirectly force us to get some exercise on the stairs. (There was no one at anytime seeing to it that the schedule she set for us was carried out. A person had to want to get well, and be motivated from within in order to apply themselves to her routine.)

Another interesting rule—no one wears shoes in the house. There are beautiful hardwood floors and she believes that the exercise is good for the feet as well as believing in the idea that it is good for the feet to be as close to the ground as possible. It took awhile to get used to going barefoot, and much longer to get used to climbing to the fourth floor and back down. For me, the latter was a very real effort. I gradually grew accustomed to it.

No one there was to be taking any medication of any kind. This eliminated my autogenous vaccine, the BCG, the gamma globulin, the vitamins and the food supplements. I couldn't help but wonder, "Am I signing my own death warrant? Can I get back on these fast enough if this doesn't work?"

Although there was much fear and trepidation connected with giving up all these possible "helps," there was also a tremendous psychological release in not having to bother with something that didn't seem to be working for me anyway. Then the question popped into my mind, "Am I trading bondage to one thing for another?" That remained to be seen.

Ann also requested that there be no smoking in the house and no television. She feels that people come to learn, and she wants to give them every opportunity to do just that. She has also recognized the possibility of the body absorbing the harmful rays from the T.V. screen.

Our room was a corner room overlooking a famous old theatre in the business section of town. We could watch the marquee change as the days went by. Living green plants kept us company and made it a warm and inviting room.

A marvelous corner bay window and another one on the front gave us a commanding view of the life on the street below. One unusual thing that we observed from these enchanting windows (or at least we thought that it was unusual at first) was that there must be either a lot of fires in Boston, a lot of false alarm fires, or a lot of practice runs for the fire engines; certainly more fires than any other place we've ever been. The fire engines seemed to run at least every thirty minutes all night long every night going somewhere.

We live in the country where the night life is very quiet except for the howling of an occasional coyote. In Boston, if we couldn't sleep at night (and I had difficulty that first night) we could sit up and watch the fire engines! However, after the first evening, the fascination with fire engines cooled down, and it wasn't long before I learned to tune them out entirely.

We were instructed that the bedding was in the cabinet down the hall and that everyone did their own housekeeping, including caring for the plants. Student volunteers cleaned the halls and the rest of the house and probably would have cleaned our room for a small fee, but I rather enjoyed doing it myself.

One area where we felt that we were extremely fortunate was in the fact that we had a bathroom with our room. Many of the others had to use common baths down the hall. When we got into the routine of taking the enemas and the implants of wheatgrass juice, we were really grateful that we didn't have to adjust our schedule to someone else's.

The furniture was of the same ancient period as the mansion. It bore no resemblance to the modern hotels and motels that we Americans know so well. Nothing was plush. It was like stepping back into old-time Boston, and somehow the old-fashioned atmosphere and the simplicity of it all was refreshing and homey.

Now it was easier to understand why it was only costing us $90.00 a week (in 1973).

It wasn't long before we had met all the other residents. They certainly were a congenial group and came from all walks of life. There were others like ourselves, there to try to find a way to overcome an illness that had not succumbed to conventional methods. Some were perfectly healthy and strictly students there to learn about nutrition. Before we left, we felt so very much a part of one big family that we still correspond with some of them.

OUR SCHEDULE

We were given a paper when we entered which gave us the routine to be followed.

One of the guests, a professional secretary, had had difficulty understanding the instruction sheet when she arrived and had taken it upon herself to work on a revised edition. She and Arn put their heads together and clarified the instructions for the mansion before we left.

Everybody took up different helpful jobs as the days went on.

Arn had decided to do everything that I had to do. This did make it easier for me, as it really was a heavy schedule and his companionship encouraged me.

We rose at 6:00 A.M. each morning in order to get everything done in a day. Sometimes it was a real race.

First thing we went barefoot downstairs to the kitchen to cut our own wheatgrass. (I will tell you more about the wheatgrass later as it plays a very definite role in my recovery.) Then we ground our wheatgrass so that it became a juice and returned to our room.

Time then to take an enema, then an implant with the wheatgrass juice. The implant was done with a catheter tube inserted on the end of the hose to the enema container, in place of the standard nozzle. The catheter tube is about 18 inches long and 3/16 of an inch in diameter and was inserted all the way up into the bowel. It didn't hurt. I couldn't even feel it, apparently there are no nerves in the bowels. Once the wheatgrass juice had been placed in the bowel, the tube was removed, then one was supposed to hold the wheatgrass juice for fifteen or twenty minutes. This places the wheatgrass juice in a spot where it migrates into your system, but holding it there for this long was something else. After much experimentation, some of it discouraging, and much of it laughable, I found that the best way for me to hold it was to scoot up the wall with my feet up. (Now you know all my secrets.)

Next came exercise class between 7:00 and 8:00 A.M. We did light exercises such as stretching then relaxing, bending over a few times then relaxing, three or four sit-ups then relaxing, more like Yoga than Jack La Lanne. I was amazed at how good I felt after these exercises. They didn't take a lot of energy.

There was one dear lady who stopped the whole class several times to tell us very slowly, all the time enunciating very distinctly every syllable, exactly why she wasn't doing her exercises the way we were being instructed to do them. She had quite a mind of her own, as well as a will to have everyone know exactly what she was thinking on every subject, with absolutely no manners whatever about interrupting others. I confess I wasn't unhappy when her time was up and she departed.

One little old man, eighty years old, delighted in spending his time in exercise class standing on his head. He was in good health. He just liked the place and had come for a vacation. After carefully attending all the classes on nutrition, and seemingly enjoying the raw fruit and raw vegetable diet that we were on, he would stop by a local drugstore and buy and eat candy bars on his afternoon walk. Sugar and candy were "no-no's." One way or another, he would add comedy to our days.

Breakfast came next. We all fixed our own with the old-timers showing the newcomers how to prepare the food and how to juice the wheatgrass. Everybody was helpful. We were promptly instructed that the first three days were a time for cleansing our systems, and the only thing we would be eating for the next three days would be watermelon (juiced) because it was in season. Other fruits were used as they came in season. An old-timer showed us how to cut it up and put it through the juicer. How would you like a half a watermelon for breakfast? I eat it often now.

Lecture classes were attended after breakfast. The classes were usually taught by Ann's paid helpers. We learned a lot about the preparation and combining of raw foods, enzymes in "live" food (anything raw, seeds, nuts, etc.), how cooking destroys enzymes (important to cancer people because they have a digestive problem especially with protein, and enzymes are needed in order to digest food), how to grow wheatgrass and sprouts, and why we should eat certain foods. There were classes both morning and afternoon all on related topics. It was like being back in school again.

We checked the bulletin board in the dining room everyday to see what classes were scheduled (generally there were special lecturers invited in on Sunday evenings). I remember one lecture on acupuncture, one on helpful pressure techniques (or as some put it "needleless acupuncture"), and one on the proper mental attitude for healing. We took the opportunity one evening to go to a meeting in an auditorium in Boston to hear a lecture on mind-control which kept us out past our 10:00 P.M. bedtime. Trying to sneak in around midnight without disturbing anyone else, we were caught red-handed by Ann Wigmore who was scrubbing the kitchen floor of all things. She didn't miss much.

Following the morning class, it was time for another wheatgrass implant. After awhile I had the feeling that fifty percent of the implants were missed by some of the people. We were determined to give Ann Wigmore's theories every chance to prove themselves, so we did not miss even one of them. With us, it was a matter of life or death.

GETTING TO KNOW ANN WIGMORE

If we stayed on schedule, we'd have about a half hour before lunch to take a walk, sometimes to a laundromat, sometimes down the tree-planted center lane of Commonwealth Avenue, but we always made it back for lunch because this was when Ann was available for questions.

Years ago in Lithuania, Ann Wigmore's grandmother had been a practical doctor. This trait was certainly inherited by Ann. She is very much of an individualist, genuinely pleasant and friendly, and a very practical person. The proof of the pudding was whether it worked or not. Her theories did not come out of a test tube in the laboratory, but out of the test tube of practical experience, although she has taken her wheatgrass, rejuvelac, and sprouts to a number of scientists and had them tested in many ways.

She stayed very busy on the fifth floor with her writing and correspondence. She never doctored. Her only purpose in the school is to teach dietetics and nutrition (all about raw foods, why they help, and how to prepare them). She is an excellent teacher.

Ann always said grace before each meal and is a firm believer in the Almighty, with a very real faith in straight thinking. She was there every lunch hour for a question and answer period during which time she would often show us something valuable about growing things, or about nutrition, or about preparing foods.

One day Ann showed us how to open a coconut properly. She pointed out the three eyes at the end of the coconut, took a screwdriver and found the soft eye, then poked it out to get the milk. Then she put the coconut into a plastic bag and whacked it good with a hammer. This way the coconut doesn't fly all over the kitchen. All the pieces end up neatly inside the bag.

Letters from old students who kept Ann posted as to how they were getting along were often shared with us at dinner. At mealtimes, discussions could range anywhere from someone telling of a better way to peel an artichoke to natural beauty aids.

Ann had a publication she was putting out, literature relative to health and religion. One Saturday afternoon we counted, bundled, and tied all the packages for mailing out her publication. Everyone was expected to be part of the family and help with these odd jobs.

The dining room was very friendly but different. There were beautiful flowers around the table and at one end of the room in a large window she had several big racks holding trays filled with growing bean sprouts, wheatgrass, and sunflower seed sprouts. Plants were hanging in the windows and it all looked very inviting.

With so many green plants all around—plants in our bedrooms—plants in the halls—plants in the dining room—plants in the living areas—there were no bad odors anywhere. There was never any grease or smoke smell from the kitchen, just fresh fruit and vegetables being prepared. Everything was fresh smelling and the aroma was definitely noticeable when you walked in the house.

The thing we learned the fastest was to sit at the middle of the table. If a person sat at one end, and the food started at the other end, one just might end up with an empty plate. It was hard to have enough food for that many people.

Part of the routine was to learn how to prepare the food firsthand in the kitchen, so everybody entered in and sliced potatoes or whatever and even washed dishes after meals with the volunteers.

Ann had open house at least once or twice a week at which time many of the neighbors enjoyed dinner with us. Those evenings (very enjoyable ones by the way) we made sure that we got to dinner on time. My appetite was improving every day.

We had thought that we would have plenty of time to read and rest, but this simply was not so for we made some lasting friendships and enjoyed a number of adventures beyond the walls of the mansion. The days were very busy even after we became old-timers.

Regular attendance at all the classes was a discipline we had promised ourselves, and attend classes regularly we did. If we were going to fly three thousand miles from the west to the east coast in an attempt to gain a reprieve from the death sentence handed down to us by the cancer specialist, we figured we were not going to miss anything that would help. Sometimes when I was busy giving myself an implant, I would wonder how we had ever decided to try this way, it was almost unreal. For two weeks we "did everything that Ann Wigmore said to do" and we gained a real education on her whole procedure.

HAVING OUR FIRST COLONIC

One of the more memorable adventures that we had in Boston came about from a recommendation that Ann Wigmore made.

I've already explained that the first three days were to be a time of cleansing the whole body from within. Eating watermelon only for those first three days wasn't torture enough. I was sure that I would starve to death and not even be able to stand on my feet after this ordeal, but strangely enough I not only survived, but I suffered no loss of energy, although I have to admit my energy had been at a pretty low ebb when I began. Arn was a better gauge for this, and his energy remained high.

Ann's recommendation was that sometime during those first three days everyone was to have a colonic (a high colon irrigation) to aid in the cleansing process. There was a certain amount of mystery and dread connected with this since neither Arn nor I had ever had a colonic, nor did we even know exactly what one was, nor did I really care to find out—but I did.

Since we were given several choices as to where we could go to have the colonic, rather than just walk a few blocks which would have been very convenient, we decided to take a subway ride to the outskirts of Boston and get acquainted with more of the area.

A Mr. Sullivan had colonic equipment in an office in his home, just beyond the end of the subway, and he would meet anyone at the subway who made an appointment and requested it, then would transport them back to his office. We made our appointment with him.

There was a black woman, Viola, staying at the mansion who really wasn't ill, but she was there for the purpose of learning what she could from Ann about nutrition. She intended to pass all the knowledge that she gained at the mansion on to her people. She asked if she could go along with us when we went for the colonic, so there were three of us.

The first few miles of the subway were underground and uneventful, but suddenly the open sky came rushing in as the train broke out into the sunlight and we could see the beautiful, lush, green, tree-lined back yards along with the old Boston homes. Our home in the southwest is in the wide-open spaces of Southern California where there are very few deciduous trees, mostly eucalyptus and evergreens which give an entirely different feeling to the countryside in contrast to the dense greenery of the trees in the northeast. The leaves were just beginning to turn color and our little excursion developed into a memorably beautiful ride. We were so glad we had chosen to explore.

Viola was part of a group doing extensive work in training blacks for teaching various things, nutrition being one of them. She painted a glowing picture about how they are advancing themselves in a self-sufficient manner, providing work and other amenities for their people, training them not to depend upon government handouts but to stand on their own two feet. Our time together was very enjoyable as well as informative.

Boston was one big bag of surprises for us. Mr. Sullivan picked us up in an open convertible. Viola had on a blue and white uniform with a hood, so she was better prepared than I was. I quickly tied a handkerchief around my head and soon handkerchief and hair were flapping gayly in the breeze as we drove through the countryside to Mr. Sullivan's home.

There were some people there ahead of us, so instead of waiting inside we took a walk down by the small lake that was about two blocks away and had a little time where we could smell the sweet grasses, enjoy the warmth of the sunshine, and really visit the countryside. On the lake ducks were leisurely paddling and floating around and people were fishing. It was a setting of real tranquility, serenity, and beauty. Since architecture has always been an interest of ours, the picturesque homes around the lake were a delightful study. We could have stayed for hours.

By the time we walked back, it was getting near lunchtime and Mr. Sullivan's wife was baking homemade bread. That heavenly aroma was everywhere. For two days and one morning we had been on a watermelon juice diet, and when Mrs. Sullivan offered us her homemade bread, it almost made us break our vows, but somehow we managed to withstand the temptation. Arn laughingly recounted later that he had had the fight of his life to keep from touching that homemade bread. That first week on Ann's diet took all of our will power.

Our fears of the unknown "colonic" proved to be unfounded as it was less uncomfortable than taking an enema. The colonic rectal speculum (the inserting tube) is a single tube that is inserted into the rectum which has two rubber tubes extending from it. One tube is attached to the incoming water supply and the other is attached to the outflow of the bowel content so that there is a constant inflow outflow through the mechanism of the machine. The water is warmed to body temperature or slightly warmer depending upon the comfort of the patient. The pressure of the inflow outflow is also controlled. This water irrigates the bowel and the waste material and toxins are carried out simultaneously while the patient is very comfortably lying down. It is not unpleasant at all. (According to a conversation I had with one doctor, this method helps to improve liver function also.)

Mr. Sullivan, a retired fireman, was very proficient at his trade and to top it all off, he gave us a very thorough and relaxing massage afterwards. Add a shower to this and I assure you that I have never been cleaner inside and outside at the same time in all my life.

Having been on our diet a few days, our systems had already begun to lose the toxicity that we had had before. Then with the colonic, the massage, and the shower, we left feeling like brand new people and several pounds lighter...just great.

One adventure wasn't enough for one day. When we got back to the mansion, it was time for our wheatgrass juice. Arn's experimental nature got the best of him. Since a little wheatgrass juice is supposed to be good for you, he figured that a lot would be even better. Being terribly rich, wheatgrass juice is a little hard to get down. I promptly got sick from drinking mine. He bravely decided that he would show me how it's done. So he took five ounces in one sitting with no other food to help absorb it. There wasn't another thing in his stomach as he had just been cleaned out as thoroughly as anyone could possibly be. He had had no warning as to what would happen, but what did happen was that about fifteen minutes later, Arn fairly floated down the stairs and had a hard time negotiating the sidewalk. For about an hour he was high on wheatgrass. (Have a glass of grass!) In that comedy hour, we learned how *not* to take wheatgrass. The old-timers laughed the loudest of all.

We had missed a meal with our trip to outer Boston, so we made up for it with extra watermelon at the evening meal. Wouldn't you know that they had sauerkraut (a favorite of ours) for dinner that evening! After resisting homemade bread at noon, then sauerkraut for dinner, I felt that someone should have pinned medals on us for good behavior. That was our last day on strictly watermelon and I heaved a sigh of relief. The next day (raise the flag) we were able to start on the same food that the old-timers were having.

The world is full of wonderful people and Hazel is one of them. She came to the mansion frequently and helped out in the kitchen after spending hours in the health food store that she owned. She sold wheatgrass that she grew, all kinds of sprouts that she sprouted and ice cream that she made from soybeans, as well as, many other delectible items. Hazel had made the sauerkraut and bless her soul, she saved some for us to eat the following evening. In fact, near the end of our two weeks when it was almost time for us to go home, she made a special trip and brought us some more.

During the second week of our stay in Boston, we became old-timers. We found that the classes repeated themselves about every ten days and we began to feel like we could spare a little more time to stretch our wings.

OTHER FOND MEMORIES OF BOSTON

In the course of a lifetime many people cross the path of one person. Many we forget almost as fast as we brush against them, while some become a vital part of our lives and even after we've parted from them, live on in our memories.

There was one couple in Boston whom we'll never forget, Paul and Magdalen. Magdalen volunteered occasionally at the mansion and helped out in the kitchen. We became acquainted one evening when her husband, Paul, who was a police officer nearing retirement, stopped to pick up Magdalen. He had walked a beat in his early days with the Boston Police Force, but now had an inside office job. Although our backgrounds are very different, and our occupations miles apart, a spontaneous friendship began to grow. Being on the police force, he had irregular hours, so occasionally had an afternoon or morning free. A number of times Magdalen and Paul invited us to go along with them (and we went) to see more of Boston and the surrounding area.

We enjoyed going with Paul and Magdalen to the Flea Market nearby in downtown Boston. It was a treat to browse among the antiques. To get into the area we had to pay an admission. The streets were roped off and there were little booths on each side. As we got further into the market, booths were set up in the streets as well, with people selling all kinds of handmade items as well as antiques; in many ways it was similar to the craft fairs in Old Town, San Diego, California.

We browsed through all kinds of artifacts, dishes, statues, etc. and came away with a few "treasures": an antique dish, several small platters, and a gold coin. I had been interested in having a gold coin that had my birthdate on it and lo and behold, there it was in the Flea Market in Boston, Massachusetts. My day was made.

Other side trips that Paul and Magdalen engineered were: an interesting visit to the old Heinz Pickle family residence where a religious school is being started; a walk along the Atlantic Ocean shore north of Boston where we were able to admire the old homes and the architecture of that day; a stop or two in a few small towns along the ocean where we inspected things like lobster traps firsthand; a visit to their own home, one of the old Boston row houses; and, knowing of our interest in organic gardening, Paul took us to some greenhouses in Boston where we had a good time talking with and learning from the men in charge.

On our own, we also found a few favorite jaunts. One was down to the old residential section of Boston called Knob Hill (I understand that there was a day when this was better known as Snob Hill). It amazed me that the flavor of old Boston has been maintained to this day. There are still gas head street lights, the original decor, and each little balcony has a flower box.

Along the same route there were many antique shops and woodworking shops down below the sidewalk level. We had to walk down three or four steps to get in and look around. Although there were beautiful things to look at, I just browsed because their prices were too high. Antiques are more expensive in Boston than in California—sorry about that, Boston—with the exception of the Flea Market where prices were good.

At times it almost seemed like we were walking through a museum as we walked and explored those old back streets.

We discovered a health food store which was designed very similarly to an old general store. It had all kinds of grains, beans and produce in old wooden barrels with scoops and sacks where the customer helped himself. They had a large variety of things, but we, adhering strictly to our diets, curbed our desire and simply enjoyed walking through and admiring.

If anyone had told us the first evening when we were considering flying east to Ann Wigmore's mansion, that before our two weeks were up, we would feel that we had had some vacation thrown in with our march against death, I don't think that we would have believed them. No question about it, we had.

THE TURNING POINT

Looking back on these episodes, I think that the significant factor to be noted was that without consciously thinking about it, we had arrived at a mental condition where we were able to enjoy other things again rather than doting on cancer and my physical problems.

Somewhere in that second week we began to feel that we were going to win the battle.

We had begun to believe in what we were doing. We had begun to feel that Ann Wigmore just might be on the right track with her "live" food theories. Boston was my turning point, the start of my recovery. I knew that something was happening, I could feel it.

In the beginning of the two weeks at the mansion, Arn had had to literally drag me at times to get me through the schedule, it was such an effort. Now I was keeping up with him fairly well, not that all my energy had returned by a long shot, but I had gained some and I knew it.

I had lost twenty-eight pounds from the time of surgery, this still concerned me, but Arn had lost ten pounds since we had arrived in Boston so I didn't feel quite so bad as I might have otherwise.

It did seem like my lumps were a little bit smaller. Maybe that was my desire more than reality, I'm not sure. I had not had the lumps removed, and I still haven't. We decided to use them as our indicators. This way we could tell whether we were on the right track. They have proved to be very valuable.

As we were leaving at the end of our two weeks, Ann came down to send us off in her own sweet way. She tucked big bags of wheatgrass under our arms to carry us over until we got ours started at home, and passed on a little more of her wisdom which is typically her:

> "Remember that your success is enhanced by your own positive inner convictions and attitudes. By keeping them on a high level, you are cooperating with Mother Nature to the fullest, creating the proper environment for healing and rejuvenation to take place. Here's to more vibrant health, greater awareness and self-fulfillment as you embark on your new adventure into the study and use of 'Living Foods.'"

The hopeful signs of the beginning of my recovery made Arn and me decide to put into practice in our regular daily living routine everything we had learned in those two weeks. It was going to mean many changes in our daily lives, but we both had the conviction that it was right for us.

We climbed aboard the airplane trying not to look like a couple of hayseeds, not the least bit embarrassed, but rather enjoying the curious and questioning glances at our wheatgrass. I began to realize how many questions I would be answering in the coming months.

The stewardess assured us that not long after we were off the ground, she would be bringing us a nice steak dinner and coffee. She appeared somewhat taken aback when we replied, "No thank you, we will just eat our apples."

We had begun a new way of life.

5

OUR NEW ADVENTURE IN USING "LIVING FOODS"

FROM EAST TO WEST

Fear had been my constant companion on our way east. Now upon our return home, I was still scared but with a difference. I know that I had experienced some kind of reversal because the lumps had not grown any larger, and might even be a little smaller. We rejoiced in new found hope.

Now we had the challenge of figuring out how we could manage a "living foods" diet in our old surroundings. It was going to be a very different kind of life.

So many questions and ideas were popping into my mind! What would our children, Arn's parents and our friends think? Would they think that we had gone overboard—too far out? Would we be labeled health food "nuts"? It was one thing to answer questions from strangers, and another to face our loved ones with a whole new way of life.

What would I serve when we had company for dinner? Well, Ann Wigmore had guests several times a week and they seemed to enjoy it! Her guests had chosen to come knowing what was in store for them. I guess I could tell any guests what I had in store for them! How could I accept an invitation to dinner?

But it doesn't really matter does it? I am alive and I am beginning to feel a little better...still scared, yes, and apprehensive about having to explain our new habits, but maybe the challenge will be good for me. It will be something to think about besides how I am feeling.

In fact, now that I think about it, it could be a whole new exciting adventure to teach others (that want to learn) a healthful way of living and eating. Surely we are not meant to have this knowledge stop right here with us. How great that Viola, our black friend is returning to teach her people.

Maybe someday I can even write a book so that many more people will have the chance to learn what we have been taught. There are so many people despondent because of cancer . . . without hope. Perhaps they can be helped by my experience. Well, I had better concentrate on making this thing work for me before trying to help others.

A NEW WAY OF SHOPPING

Our first stop on our way home from the airport was our favorite fruit and farm produce stand "Takahashi." We took home five watermelons, a crate of oranges, a rack of bananas, pounds of carrots, celery, cucumbers, parsley, tomatoes, green peppers, corn on the cob and all kinds of squash. The owners of the stand were delighted. Over the next few weeks and months we developed a real rapport with them as we bought larger and larger orders of fruits and vegetables.

When we shared my problem with them, and the intricacies of the "living foods" diet, they were not only cooperative, but seemed to be very interested in learning about the fruit and vegetable combinations that complement each other. When they knew what we needed, they put aside items for us that were hard to acquire other places. It has been our experience that people have wanted to help us all they can.

Today, my trips to the supermarket are not for food. I bring home a case of paper towels, a case of toilet paper, half a dozen bottles of distilled water, (for Arn's batteries and my iron) and a half a dozen bottles of white vinegar (my cleaning agent) and only need to go about every three months.

LESSONS WE LEARNED IN
OUR GARDEN

The first few days of our return from Ann Wigmore's were upside down. Trying to get ourselves organized into a routine that allowed us to keep our Boston schedule, (remember Arn had decided to continue on the "living foods" with me) catching up on jobs undone around the house for the two weeks we'd been gone and Arn working in the office full time, made it a furious pace crowding every minute of every day with things that needed to be done, all of them right now.

Getting some wheatgrass started was the first "must," then we started some sprouts. Rather than shop everyday for fresh fruits and vegetables, Arn designed, and we built comparatively inexpensively, a walk-in cooler room. We decided to grow our own food so that we could have it available year-round, so next came the greenhouse. It was a major undertaking which turned out to be a really fun job. We bought a kit and every minute that we were free during the following three weeks were spent getting the greenhouse put together. It's a beauty, measuring fourteen feet by twenty-two feet and worth every bit of three weeks of hard labor.

One real drawback to our plans was the fact that our soil was very poor. A time of trial and error followed with our trying many different things to make our soil nutritious. We finally decided to go the organic way. This meant that we could not fertilize the soil in our greenhouse with chemical fertilizers (which would have given us the most rapid growth.). So our first real try at growing was slow, but from our research we had decided the organic way seemed to be the most natural and the most fruitful in the long run.

We invested in worms. They had to be bought and transplanted into the soil. Can you imagine soil so poor that it didn't even have worms? That was ours. I never dreamed that I could ever become attached to earthworms, but I have. These little fellows work day in and day out just for us, continually digging up the ground, and making it better than it was before.

I learned that they digest the soil, actually eating and conditioning it. To an important extent, our topsoils have practically been made by earthworms. That is why Aristotle called them the intestines of the soil. Their castings are far richer minerally than the soil which they ingest. It is said that an average earthworm will produce its weight in castings every twenty-four hours. They burrow into the ground, as far as six feet down, aerating the soil, making holes for rain to penetrate. They break up hardpans. Each year their dead bodies furnish a considerable amount of valuable nitrogenous fertilizer, which may amount to more than a thousand pounds per acre in a highly "organic soil."[1]

Noted earthworm researcher Charles Darwin found that the amount of soil these creatures pass through their bodies annually can be as much as fifteen tons of dry earth an acre. In so doing, the digestive juices of the earthworm make the soil's organic matter and mineral content more valuable to plants. These are a few other reasons why earthworms are rated so highly.[2]

With our increasing abundance of worms, I began to wonder if they would harm the plants themselves. No need to worry, the worms do not eat living plants, they eat only dead material. I think they have been to all of Ann Wigmore's classes and as a consequence know exactly what not to eat! If any of the plants are left in the ground long enough to decay and rot, the worms immediately begin to eat them until there is nothing left.

I would guess that there are no limits to the amount of worms you could have. However, I would imagine that if you couldn't feed them fast enough, they wouldn't propagate. Earthworms are bi-sexual, with both male and female reproductive organs; each earthworm is capable of producing egg capsules, but must first have contact with another worm to be fertilized. Their eggs hatch in about twenty-one days. [3]

We have become very sentimental and protective towards the worms because they are constantly saving us the problem of shovelling and keeping the soil loose in the greenhouse. Now our soil is continually getting better. We learned to use organic matter, like carrot tops, that usually is wasted. Instead of throwing them away, we throw them on the ground in the greenhouse and with our abundance of worms, within two or three days they are taken into the ground. We take all the pulp from our juicer, (learned from Ann Wigmore) and any vegetable matter that has been ground up fine and scatter it around in the greenhouse everyday to feed the worms. We see to it that they are well fed and they in turn see to it that our soil becomes richer and richer.

Since Arn's work schedule did not allow much time for gardening we had to streamline our greenhouse so that it did most of the work for us. We put in a semi-automatic watering system and made the heating completely automatic. We were very pleasantly surprised to find that both of us thoroughly enjoy the work in the greenhouse. There is something very satisfying about producing our own food. It is a continuing adventure.

In times past, we had tried to raise a garden with very little success. The rabbits, the deer and other predators always knew exactly when we planted. I'm relatively sure they thought we were planting for them, because as soon as something came up through the ground they helped themselves and never left anything for us. Our beautiful greenhouse eliminated this problem.

We hung a big sign on the door of the greenhouse, "Garden of Eydie—No rabbits, no deer or other predators allowed," and evidently they can read!

As our soil became physically, chemically and biologically sound with the help of our worm friends, our greenhouse became a thing of great joy.

At first we grew our wheatgrass in the greenhouse in trays; then we decided to splurge and build special racks which we attached to the sides of the greenhouse. Now these racks hold all of our sprouting wheatgrass trays without usurping valuable garden space.

We have another friend in our greenhouse who works for us everyday at least eight hours, perhaps more. He doesn't believe that he needs a union card in order to get fair treatment. In fact, he even enjoys working overtime free...Mr. Friendly Toad. He cleans up all the bugs. At least, I always blame it on him because our greenhouse is pest free! I never cease to be amazed at the lack of pests.

Even on cold days, it is warm in our greenhouse. Invisible rays filter through the cloud layers and warm up the greenhouse, and of course, the greenhouse itself protects everything growing inside from the winds. We have an abundance of tomatoes, carrots, radishes, onions, celery, beets, several kinds of lettuce, comfrey, parsley, mint, green and red peppers, nasturtiums, pansies, and we even start plants for transplanting.

We decided that we wanted to eventually produce all the food that we eat to insure that it is all organically grown without any sprays or poisons. We planted fifty fruit trees around the property, of various kinds that we felt would give us year-round supply. Unfortunately, it will take at least five years before they produce enough to supply all our needs, so our farm produce stand still gets a lot of business from us.

From what we have read and studied, we are in agreement with those who consider the organic way the best for growing fruit trees. We feed the fruit trees with garbage, then cover the garbage with straw. This gets watered-in slowly by using a drip irrigation method which takes the nutrients into the ground and prevents the material from washing away. We also transplanted worms around the trees to help in this process.

Our trees are already bearing fruit, not a lot but they are giving us by far the most delicious fruit that we have ever tasted, especially when there is only one on a tree. I'm sure that there is something psychological about that, but it's fun anyway. I've heard someone say that when you grow your own, it's got to be good whether it is or not (but ours really is!).

One more shortcut that we are employing is mulching. This is a slightly different method for outside gardening. Author Ruth Stout describes it in her "No Work Garden Book." It is almost as revolutionary a way of gardening as the nutritional approach is to conquering cancer. She has figured out a way of gardening which brings top results with a minimum of labor. There is no weeding and no plowing. She uses all kinds of organic matter, especially hay, straw, spoiled hay, and leaves, spreading it thickly over the entire garden except, of course, on top of the seeds that she plants. Within a couple of years she found she was able to abandon all commercial fertilizers. After spreading the straw around, she found that the only jobs left were planting, thinning, and the picking. Whenever she wants to put in some more seeds, she pulls the mulch back and plants. Later, when the seeds have sprouted, she pulls the mulch close around the little plants, thus keeping the ground around them moist and outwitting the weeds.

I knew that I had to try her method when she suggested that I hunt up a secondhand store and get rid of my hoes and spades and cultivators; that the largest digging tool I would need would be a trowel.

We have found her theories to be very sound through our own practical experience. We do not turn the soil or weed. We utilize earthworms and let nature do the work. We keep a heavy mulch of straw on the garden and the weeds never get enough light to draw their heads up. The nutrients are continually going back into the soil as the material decays, thus we have continuous fertilization. The mulch covering the ground prevents moisture from escaping so there is either no watering at all or a greatly reduced watering program. In our dry territory in Southern California, the conservation of water is greatly appreciated.

Conservation of time...conservation of water...it is working for us.

WHAT ABOUT MY CANCER

About three weeks had lapsed while we were getting ourselves straightened out at home, in the office and in the garden (getting our wheatgrass started and our greenhouse finished). It was time to revisit my doctor.

Remember, we had not told the doctor yet that we had gone to Boston. I went through the usual routine of tests. When the report came in from my tests this time, the doctor saw a change. We were informed that the urine colony count had gone from 300 down to 120. There may have been other favorable indications but I don't remember them because the doctor was so full of questions.

The fear that had been my daily companion since the first lump had been found, finally found release and just faded into oblivion. The hours of wondering were over. We were making progress. My joy was unbounded!

When we told the doctor what we had done, we were assured that no matter how unorthodox the treatment might be, the doctor's interest was in curing cancer, not judging the method. After hearing it all, we were asked to write it all down...everything that was entailed in the diet...everything that we had done physically from the moment we had risen in the morning until we had gone to bed at night. The doctor wanted to study it all very carefully to try to understand what the active element was that was causing the reversal.

We came back with a lengthy written dissertation on our two weeks with Ann Wigmore at the Mansion.

As I recall, one of the doctor's first questions was, "What is wheatgrass?"

So I grew a tray of wheatgrass and took it into the doctor's office. Heretofore it had always been thought that the helpful ingredient in the wheatgrass was the chlorophyll it produced, but chlorophyll does not kill cancer cells. The doctor had to look beyond the chlorophyll. We have the utmost respect and admiration for this doctor's inquisitive research-oriented mind.

Speaking of chlorophyll and the research-mind reminds me of Mr. Charles Kettering, for many years the director of the Sloan-Kettering Institute and Chairman of the Board of the Charles S. Kettering Foundation for Researches in the Natural Sciences. He had sponsored work researching chlorophyll and cancer. We have the utmost respect and admiration for his work.

This American engineer and inventor, the same Mr. Kettering, vice-president of General Motors Corporation for 27 years and General Manager of their Research Laboratory Division, is a hero of Arn's. Arn tells me that he was a man who did not follow the book. He refused to hire anyone in his research department with more than a high school education, because the college graduates knew the book too well and Kettering wanted original ideas. His team developed many things that might never have been developed because his people did not know that they could not be done.

I'm not disparaging knowledge gleaned from books, or I wouldn't be writing a book myself. What I would like to discredit is the closed mind—closed simply because someone else said—someone else wrote—or a college professor taught—or the recognized authority on the subject says to do it this way—or because my intellectual friend says it can't be done etc. It seems to me that since the world began, new and different ideas and ways of doing things have been slowly revolutionizing society. A new way, or a natural way, or an underlying principle has always been there, but man just seems to have to slowly uncover these truths that have been there all the time. Sometimes the less formal schooling that a person has, the easier it is for him to stretch his mind.

Believe me, we had to do some mind-stretching when we started considering the idea of drinking wheatgrass juice and eating only live raw foods to bring about a reversal with my malignant breast cancer. Now we are very grateful to be in a position where we can begin to understand it from the scientific viewpoint.

Within the next year, the doctor's research uncovered the unknown ingredient that could reverse the growth of a cancerous tumor. The doctor made it known to us that it is the abscisic acid in the wheatgrass that reverses the growth. In the experimental tests abscisic acid in its natural form was found to be deadly against any form of cancer—and it takes only a very small amount. When some live tumor-bearing animals were given injections of abscisic acid, their tumors quickly deteriorated. As I understand it, this work is still in the research stages.

It would seem that the time is not too far distant when abscisic acid pills or a new vaccine will be developed from this research to halt the march of this dread disease.

By saying this, are we saying that a person will be able to scratch the wheatgrass therapy and the "living foods" diet and all that goes with it and be able to handle the cancer just with abscisic acid pills or a vaccine? Arn and I both believe that there is every possibility that this may happen.

However, poor eating habits cause more diseases than cancer. We may be able to reverse cancer with abscisic acid pills, but then die from a heart attack or something else.

As for us, we will continue with the "living foods" diet plus the wheatgrass therapy (even if a pill or vaccine is manufactured) because our health has become so extraordinarily good that we believe it is the way for the best possible health to be maintained. The importance of this at this time, of course, is that the wheatgrass is still the only way we know to obtain the natural abscisic acid in a large enough quantity to do the job for me, since it is found only in minute quantities in other live raw foods.

Ann Wigmore has said, "I am continuously receiving testimonials from individuals all over the globe who, using the wheatgrass therapy and living food, have helped to eliminate cancerous growths and other mental and physical health problems."[4]

Subsequent visits to the doctor's office revealed that my urine colony count was slowly but steadily going down. For two months it was five—two more months and it was two—then an unbelievable zero! (This was only one factor in a complex series of testing).

After awhile I began to notice things like my hair getting soft again and my nails getting flexible. For over a year I had been complaining about my hair getting coarse, blaming the shampoo, but secretly wondering if it had any further significance. Later, I discovered that a change in the texture of the hair is a sign of cancer.

Over a period of three to four months after our time in Boston, my tiredness gradually disappeared. There was a period when I would still tire more easily than I desired, but then my energy returned in full and that was a cause for rejoicing.

What a joy it was to have an appetite again, to be able to sit down and later get up rested and to wake up in the morning ready to face a new day instead of being just as aching-tired as when I went to bed.

My weight had just about returned to normal (my normal is between 104-107 lbs.).

Normal. What a marvelous word! Will I be able to live a normal life staying on my living foods diet? So far, it has meant many changes in my life, but then there is nothing constant in life but change anyway. Where will my limitations be? Our eating habits have been changed, but that's been fun, and I continue to learn in this area. When we eat out, I am limited but there is always something on the menu that I can eat. More and more we are discovering new vegetarian restaurants which makes it even easier. It's really not a problem. When friends invite us to dinner, I am simply frank about the limitations of my diet and they don't seem to mind. Their salads are just as good as mine. When visiting our family I'll take my own sandwich or fruit if they're fresh out of something for me to eat.

Would it restrict a vacation? I had begun to feel *so*

good that I thought we might be able to take a holiday and do some traveling. Going on a trip would be one way to find out how much my life was going to be limited.

Arn and I had often thought we'd like to find out for ourselves by firsthand experience whether Europe has seen any breakthrough on cancer. Perhaps the Medical Center at the University of Zurich, Switzerland would be a good place to check this out. We would go to Switzerland.

6 | TRAVEL AND "LIVING FOODS"

SWITZERLAND

Could we travel and stay on the "living foods" diet? The more we talked about it, the more we began to believe that we could do it. I was doing so well that we decided I should be able to give up the wheatgrass for a period of ten days at least, which would be long enough to enjoy a trip to Switzerland. We would stay strictly on salads, raw vegetables, raw fruits, raw nuts and seeds.

Preparing for our vacation trip was exciting and filled with pleasure. Maps have always fascinated me so we started out by getting a large detailed map of tiny little Switzerland. Soon we had all the major cities in their proper places and could begin to wonder about all the small towns. Which ones should we explore? Small towns have always been more interesting to us. It seems like a stranger can usually become better acquainted with the people of a small town than in the impersonal busyness of a metropolitan area, and we like people.

The travel brochures all looked inviting. The

hardest decision was where did we want to go? Did we want to see more by moving around a lot or be content with a few highlights, and really get to know a place and possibly a few people at the same time? We decided on the latter.

Finally we were on our magic carpet and in only a few hours were flying over some of the most magnificent mountainous country to be found anywhere in the world, the Swiss Alps.

We had left behind "just-a-sweater" weather in Southern California to face winter-bound Switzerland in December. We learned too late that if we had notified the airline three days in advance, they would have been happy to have supplied us with fruit or vegetarian meals. However, we had boarded the plane armed with a large bag of apples, so we ate apples...live and learn.

Soon we were taking colored pictures of the snow-clad Alps as they stretched in all their magnificent grandeur from one end of Switzerland to the other. If a person likes rugged mountains, I'm sure that there is no more beautiful country than this one.

ZURICH

We have a friend who loves to visit Switzerland and who is well acquainted with a fruit stand in Zurich of all places, so since Zurich was our first stop, our friend's fruit stand was the next. Imagine our surprise and delight when we found California fruits such as avocadoes, oranges, grapefruits and tangerines, as well as many other varieties of fruits and vegetables. You can better understand our inexperience as "vegetarian travelers" when you realize that when we were first planning our trip, we were thinking that we just might have to exist on a very limited diet such as raw potatoes and celery! Not so, we learned in advance from our friends. We had just never looked for fruit and vegetable stands before in our travels. We were much relieved when we actually found the abundance of fruit and vegetables for ourselves. We had been worried about having problems getting food.

Later, while becoming more knowledgeable about Zurich, we found many other small fruit stands. What an artist's dream! Most of these fruit stands exhibited their tempting wares on little wooden stands right on the sidewalks. Often an enchanting light snow would be falling on the street and on the stands, lightly packing the neat rows of lucious fruit in a bed of snow. It was not only an arresting artistic display for the eyes, but it also was a sensory delight to pick out the peaches and oranges peeking up through the snow. We never tired of marveling at this phenomenon wherever we found it.

Although we had no plans to do any actual skiing, we had selected a ski trip, at reduced rates, which included Zurich, a Volkswagen and quarters in a Guest House Inn in the village of Sempach, about an hour's drive out of Zurich. Off season, as we were, we were taking advantage of a tour put together for skiers. Our Volkswagen was presented to us in Zurich when we landed at the airport. After finding our fruit, all we had to do was learn to read the Swiss road maps and find Sempach.

SEMPACH

We had more than one surprise before we finished ten days in Switzerland, but I think one of the funniest was the astonishment of the villagers in Sempach. Staying at the Inn was part of the package trip, but we didn't find out until we got there, that the skiers never stopped at Sempach. They all went on up higher to mountain lodges close to the ski runs. It was almost as if the Swiss townspeople didn't quite know what to do with us. I think by the way they acted, we may have been the very first persons to have taken advantage of their part of the skiers' bargain.

Sempach is a marvelous little town, two blocks long, entered by driving through an archway at the bottom of a picturesque bell tower. Arn and I were the only strangers in town.

Old Switzerland built their houses wall to wall, so that the wall of one house, is the same wall of the house next door, very similar to the homes in San Francisco, but done specifically for the reason of conserving heat.

The Inn at Sempach consisted of three of these houses. Originally they had been the separate homes of the father and his two sons. By knocking out the

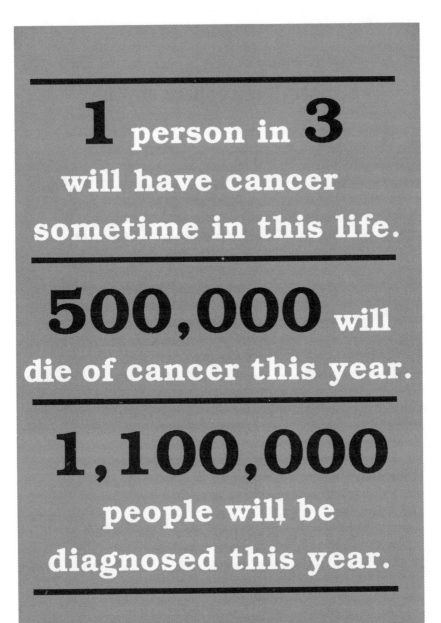

1 person in 3
will have cancer
sometime in this life.

500,000 will
die of cancer this year.

1,100,000
people will be
diagnosed this year.

As reported by the American Cancer Society, 1991

Cancer doesn't spare anyone.

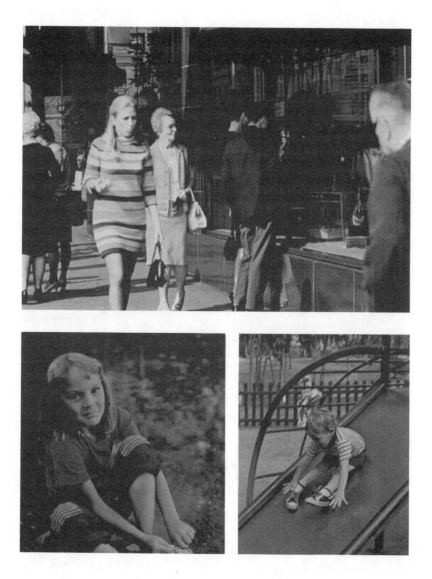

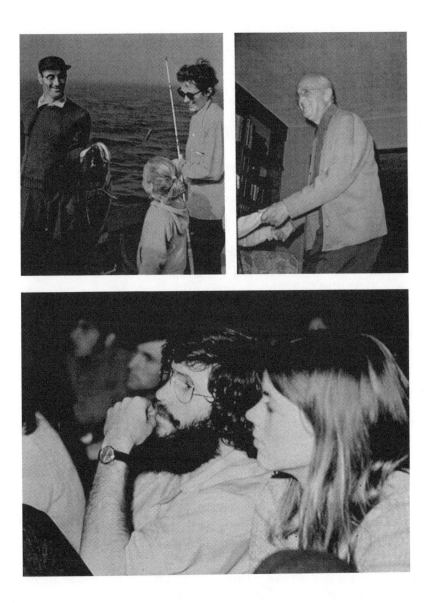

But we found an answer to cancer!

Is this at last the hoped for answer to malignant cancer?

Eydie Mae's intimate, true story reveals her daring and courageous spirit as she tells how in the face of seemingly impossible odds, she disregards the anxious concern of members of her family, and the orthodox views of her friends, and discovers a new, completely natural method of arresting cancer.

This book tells candidly how she made her decision not to have the radical mastectomy (complete removal of the breast and lymph glands by surgery) that the doctor ordered. When her husband, Arn, told the cancer specialist to cancel the operation that had been scheduled, that Eydie Mae had decided not to have the radical mastectomy the doctor had recommended, the doctor cried out in unbelief, "You are going to kill that woman!"

That was two and one-half years ago. Today, Eydie Mae is living a happy and full life, whole in body.

This is not a magic formula, but her proven practical method of overcoming cancer without surgery. In story form, she tells you step by step what she did. She also tells how because of her recovery, the substance that reverses the growth of the cancer cells has been discovered, and is now in the research stages of being tested in San Diego.

Incredible? Yes.

Impossible? No.

Eydie Mae has done it.

Also Featured Is:

- How Eydie Mae's colony count went from 300 down to zero.

- How Eydie Mae has incorporated this natural agent into her own diet.

- How Eydie Mae's malignant breast cancer brought her face to face with the reality of death, forcing her to do some real soul-searching and what she found missing.

- How Eydie Mae's soul-searching questions about life were answered, bringing new meaning and freedom into her life.

THE PUBLISHERS

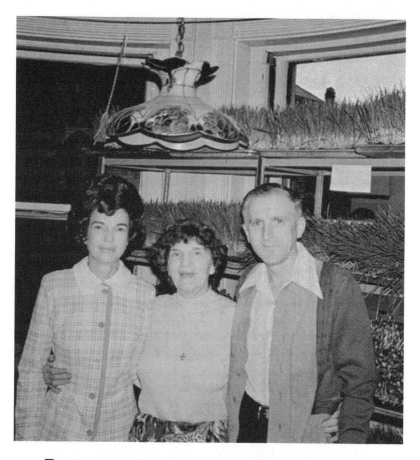

Boston—Eydie Mae, Ann Wigmore and Arn at the Hippocrates Health Institute

"Arn had had to literally drag me at times to get me through the schedule, . . . Boston was my turning point, the start of my recovery."

(See Chapter Four—The Turning Point)

The element that reverses the growth of cancer was found in wheatgrass. Wheatgrass will grow just about anywhere . . . in your garden, your kitchen or basement window, your greenhouse, or in old discarded elevators like Eydie Mae's, seen below. (See Chapter Five.)

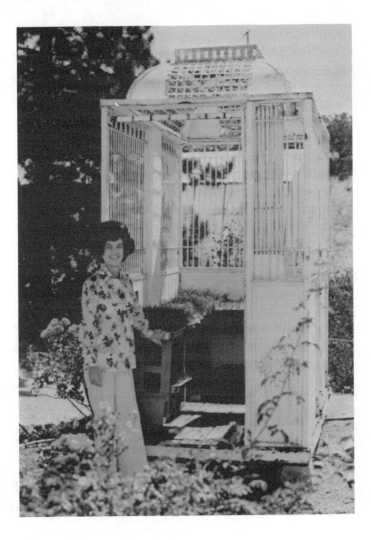

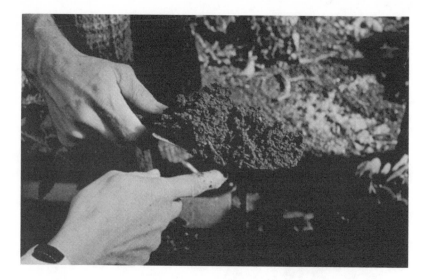

"We bought a kit to build our greenhouse...we invested in worms. Can you imagine soil so poor that it didn't even have worms? We grew our wheatgrass in trays..." (See Chapter Five.)

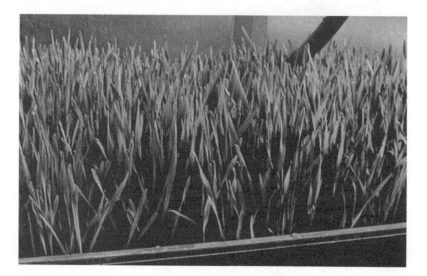

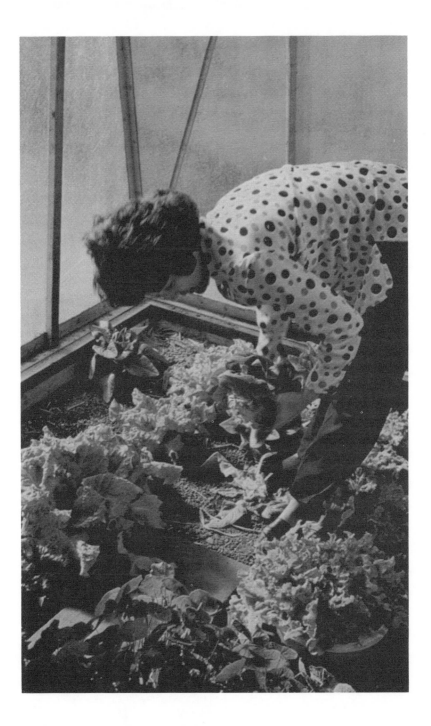

"How unbelievable! . . . here at our fingertips for so long . . . an answer to cancer . . ."

"I'm going to tell the whole world. Let them laugh at me if they want. As soon as there is no doubt in my mind at all, I'm going to shout it to the rooftops!"

"I had begun to feel so good that we decided to take a holiday in Switzerland." (See Chapter Six)

View from our room in the Inn, Sempach, Switzerland.

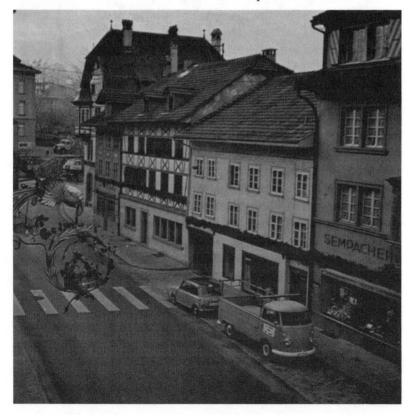

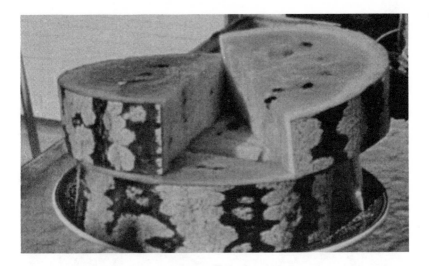

"Our trip helped me to see that I wasn't going to have to give up anything of importance because of my diet . . . No matter where we went our request for a fresh fruit meal, or a raw vegetable meal met with very little surprise and people were most helpful. It just wasn't difficult."

California Sandwich

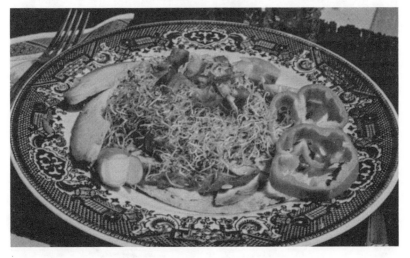

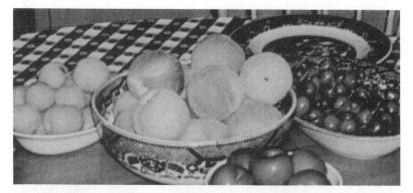

Fruit Bowl

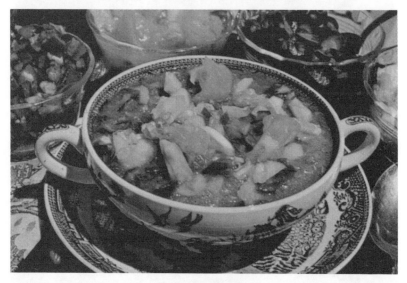

Gazpacho Soup

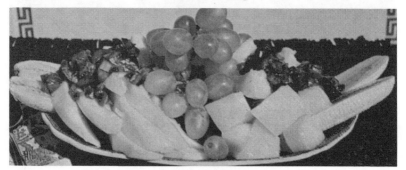

Bonanza Split

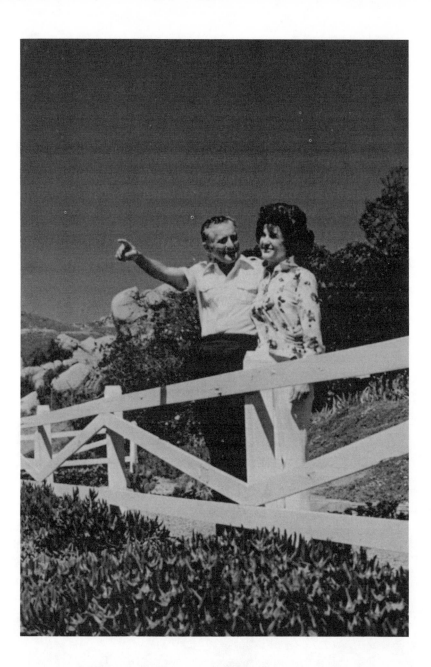

Faced with death, we found a way to live.

"Goodbye Cancer!"
The Green Cocktail
(See recipe,
Chapter 8)

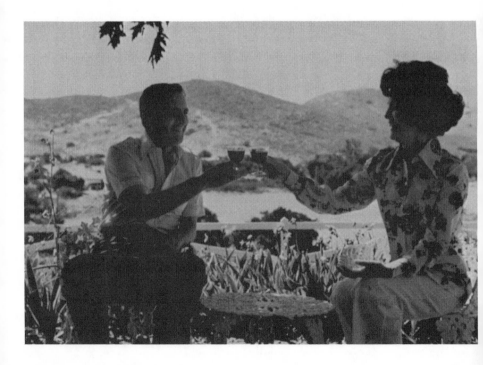

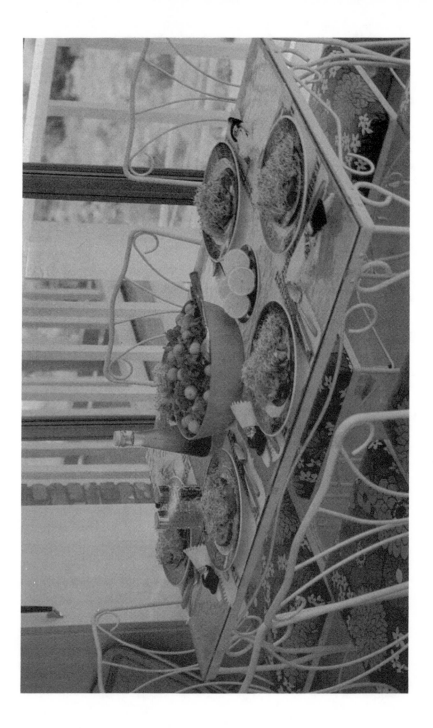

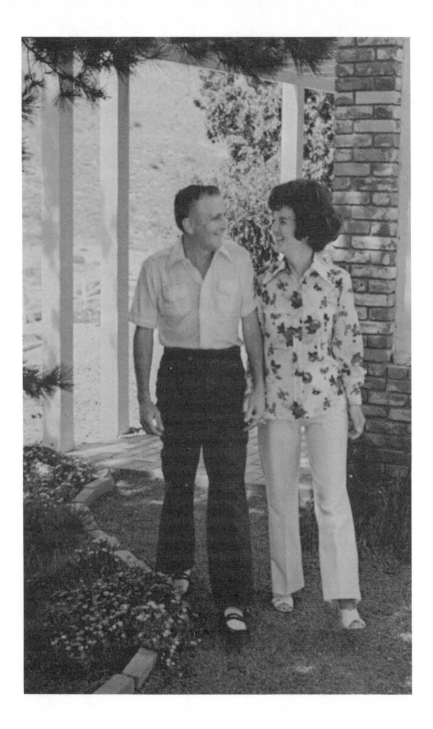

walls separating the three houses, they had built a charming inn and guest house. There was a restaurant on the second floor which doubled as the town meeting hall. It was over two hundred years old.

Our room was on the third floor with a grand view of all the activities on the street below, and the mountains in the background. The bathrooms down the hall were shared with the rest of the family. In fact, it was more like being western world relatives, than paying guests. The language barrier made us avid students of sign language.

The matron of the household spoke English well enough to be able to carry on a conversation to understand us and to make sure our needs were met. She even did a little interpreting for us. After Arn's explanation of our eating habits, she made sure that raw vegetarian meals were available any time we dined in their restaurant. She was one of the few who spoke any English in the entire village, but everyone welcomed us and made us feel at home with their ready smiles and gracious manners—very congenial people. Our sign language improved everyday.

In the wee hours of the next morning, we awakened to a clip-clop, clip-clop sound we hadn't heard before. Resisting the temptation to remain cozy and warm under our down comforter, Arn's curiosity got the best of him and he had to see what was going on down on the street. He quickly rose and cracked a window open to see. A horse-drawn milkwagon was moving slowly down the street. A word from Arn and I had to get up and see this, too. The milkman's horses were pulling a box-like trailer. It had two wheels similar to bicycle wheels attached to the sides of the box so that they extended only about two inches below the box—an ingenious contraption that enabled him to lift his milk can only a few inches to get it into the box. Where the snow had not been cleared, the box slid on top of the snow, whereas when it came to a cleared area, the box traveled on the wheels! I wanted to take a picture of this convertible sleigh, but it was too dark.

Arn promptly "blew the horn" of his Swiss ancestors, patting them on the back over this clever solution which he was sure dated from way back.

The milkman proceeded from one house to another simply dipping milk from his larger can into the smaller cans that had been left outside for this purpose. How primitive by comparison to our mechanized, motorized society in the U.S.A., and how refreshing in its simplicity! It made my heart yearn for a simpler life. Maybe there was some Swiss in me, too.

Morning was something else in Sempach. All the windows were raised as soon as the people woke up, then followed the shake down (or maybe it was a shake-up). A variety of comforters, blankets, and clothing were shaken out the windows. At times, with all those things flapping out the windows, it appeared as though the women were trying to make all the houses in Sempach take off the ground for never-never land. Huddled over our old-fashioned radiator, we watched in awe, with *our* window solidly shut, while these robust Swiss simply left their windows wide open after the shaking and the airing. It was impossible for us to imagine how these people could learn to withstand the freezing temperature, but they didn't seem to mind it at all.

We soon learned that after breakfast it was time to go to the market. Every morning all the women in town shopped for their food for the day. They didn't need to come over later for a cup of coffee and chat. They could meet every morning in the market and visit. I rather liked that too. There *must* be some Swiss in me.

I was so filled with joy one morning. My thoughts just tumbled over one another. How unbelievable! Here I am, a cancer patient, not long ago given an eighty percent chance to live one year. I'm supposed to be sick—dying, and now I'm seemingly free from all symptoms but my lumps, and they are diminishing all the time...just so long as I continue to eat live foods, and drink my wheatgrass juice. How incredible, here at our fingertips for so long, an answer to cancer!

No one will believe us.

It's too simple. It's too easy. This phantom cancer has been such a heavy, hopeless subject for so long, no one will believe us.

I don't care whether anyone believes us or not. I'm going to tell the whole world. Let them laugh at us if they want. As soon as there is no doubt in my mind at all, I'm going to shout it to the rooftops.

Oh what joy to be alive and well! Everything seems

so new and beautiful. The Bible speaks of rebirth, maybe that's like this. Everything is so three-dimensional—or is there such a thing as five-dimensional? Whatever it is, it's great! My world surely had gone flat there for awhile.

And now a vacation. There just isn't anything that I can't do, except eat certain things. Six months ago, all this would have been very hard for me to believe, but today it is all very real. It's as real as a mockingbird's song! How do I know when birds are singing? I can hear them. How would you know when my heart is singing and filled with joy? Perhaps you could hear it, too...if you were really listening. But now it's time to stop thinking and get back to our holiday in Switzerland.

After spending a little time with the Swiss road maps, we found we could get around without many problems, and took a number of side trips. One day while we were out driving, we even managed to see a baby avalanche go tumbling down one of the mountains.

BERN

Early one morning we hopped into our Volkswagen and journeyed to the beautiful city of Bern and spent a lovely day. The Swiss Republic is divided into cantons or districts. Bern, the capital of the canton of Bern and also the capital of the whole confederation is situated on an elevated Rocky peninsula washed on three sides by the Aar River, a tributary to the Rhine and the largest river in Switzerland, which is crossed by several notable bridges. The streets are adorned with many lovely fountains.

The bear is the heraldic emblem of Bern showing up frequently in sculptured form, but of more interest to me was the curious clock-tower (I love clocks) which dates back to 1527, containing a mechanism where three minutes before the hour a wooden cock crows and flaps its wings; in another minute a procession of bears passes around a seated figure of a bearded old man; the cock then crows again. The hour is struck on a bell at the top of the tower, by a figure with a hammer, and at each stroke, the bearded old man raises his sceptre and opens his mouth, while he turns an hour-glass; a bear inclines his head at the same time. Then the cock crows again. Sheer delight!

The houses were built right to the street. The second stories extended out over the sidewalks, which necessitated the building of many archways. Arn couldn't get his fill of studying the archways. He is sure that this must have been the forerunner of the malls we have today. A person could walk through the whole city without getting wet from rain or snow. Such unusual architecture. We were really impressed with the whole city.

THE UNIVERSITY OF ZURICH

Another day, we spent at the University of Zurich. This day made me realize anew how fortunate I was, a cancer patient thoroughly enjoying a vacation.

We visited their Medical Center with the express purpose of discovering whether there were any advance techniques that Europe might have in the treatment of cancer. We luckily had the opportunity to interview one of the higher authorities in the Cancer section at that time. The person we talked with was in the Chemotherapy department. She was a doctor, very cordial, who spoke English extremely well, and discussed with us in detail their use of chemotherapy. According to her, Europe had not seen any breakthrough in cancer, nor did she see anything new on the horizon. They were using the same procedures as in the United States, radical mastectomy, other surgery, etc. When the cancer progressed to a certain stage, the surgeon passed the patient on to the chemotherapy section and they picked up from there and tried to make the patient more comfortable.

She spoke of the discouragement and the heartbreak in her field of chemotherapy. Every patient that was sent to her had a death warrant. She told us that chemotherapy just wasn't used until the cancer had progressed to a certain stage; then it was just a method of retarding the growth of cancer *if* the cancer was in a vital organ. She explained that the chemotherapy does great damage to and prevents the reproduction of the healthy tissue and blood of a person's body. However, life could be prolonged with its use providing that the cancer was in a vital organ. This was the only reason that it was used, along with certain painkilling side effects. She said that if the cancer is not in a vital organ, chemotherapy should not be used. They had to be extremely careful when diagnosing because if a mistake was made, they could easily shorten a life instead of lengthening one. So hers was a job of walking a very fine line, but most difficult of all was the fact that all of her patients died. She said that the chemotherapy should never be used unless it is a terminal case. The pain of terminal cancer is very severe, a never ending, continuing pain. If her work had any saving grace, it was because the chemotherapy seemed to lessen the pain. She made the point that psychologically her job was an inordinately difficult one.

Her statistics showed that at that time in Europe, one woman in every twenty alive at that time, would be faced with breast cancer at some time in her life. Now, I understand that the statistics are somewhat worse in the United States; it's nearing one woman in fifteen.

Actually, it is a rare family today that has not been touched by this dread disease.

THE GOOSE DOWN COMFORTER

It was the third week in December and I made an

interesting note about Christmas in Switzerland. All the lights on Christmas decorations are white, tree lights included, which gives them a special beauty all their own.

A delightful surprise was in store for us on our last evening in the Inn. We had gone to bed, luxuriating in the snug warmth under our down comforter after a final day of sightseeing in our Volkswagen. I was almost asleep when suddenly live music started coming up through the floor. It was like what I imagined angel's voices from heaven would have sounded like. Then I realized it was just two days before Christmas and the choir was practicing below in the meeting hall...Oh Tannenbaum...and lovely carols. What joy! We could have listened long after they were through singing.

December in Switzerland is cold, but sleeping under their six inch thick goose down comforters is positively heavenly—weightless, warm, and wonderbar. The expression, ''snug as a bug in a rug'' must have originated under a Swiss comforter.

We liked Switzerland's answer to the electric blanket so well that we decided to find one and take it back with us to the U. S. At Jemolis' store we were faced with some fast calculations translating the comforter measurements from the metric system to American sizes, but once we picked it out, it became our prized possession. We very carefully rolled it up and hand carried it all the way back on the plane, not letting it out of our hands until we got it through the customs in New York City upon our re-entry into the States. The U. S. Customs officer looked at it with more than a suspicious eye. He poked it and punched it—then poked it and punched it again and again. It was the last thing he let go—and then reluctantly for some obscure reason. Heaven only knows what he may have thought could have been sewn inside. I had to relinquish my tangerines at customs. No fruit was allowed to enter. We finally checked our beautiful comforter through with our luggage the rest of the way to California.

Would you believe it didn't show up in San Diego? After all our painstaking care, what an unhappy letdown! You can't imagine how we had been looking forward to tearing the covers off our bed when we got home to see if it worked in the U.S.A.

Arn had carefully wrapped it in brown wrapping paper and secured a handle on it. I had written our name and address all over it, so we did go to the trouble of trying to trace it. Unbelievably, it had been shipped back to Switzerland! It did make a second trip back to the States and this time we received it. We treasure it and use it in preference to an electric blanket.

Actually, our whole ten days were packed full, with only a minimum of sleep. My energy stayed high all the way, and there seemed to be no ill effects from the trip at all.

One of the things that we learned was that our "living foods" diet was not as revolutionary as we had

originally thought. Evidently there have been vege-
tarians around for a long time that had never really
been called to our attention. No matter where we
went, our request for a fresh fruit meal, or a raw
vegetable meal met with very little surprise and
people were most helpful. It just wasn't difficult.

We have come to thoroughly enjoy eating this way
and our trip helped me to see that I wasn't going to
have to give up anything of importance because of it.

I find myself enjoying life with a greater intensity
than ever before. I've heard it said before that
sometimes our sense of appreciation for something is
newly awakened when faced with the possibility of
losing it. Whether this is the reason for my new zest
for life, or whether it is our "living foods" diet, I can't
say for sure. However, I suspect that it's related to
both things.

7

THE "LIVING FOODS" DIET

ALL OR NOTHING AT ALL

In the course of my trial by cancer, I have become acquainted with many other cancer patients. Some have accepted a few of the ideas from certain experimental programs and others have chosen a partial program in another. I have heard every variation of:
—I like this idea but I can't give up my cheese.
—I can see value in the idea, but give up chicken and eggs? I live on them.
—I'll use this portion of the diet but certainly not that.
—I could not give up coffee or leave sugar alone.
—My job requires a lot of energy so I have to have my protein, I could not give up meat. Maybe you have that kind of will power, but not me.
This latter statement about meat always reminds me of a story I heard once about a farmer who while out plowing a field with his horse stopped long enough to talk to a friendly neighbor by the fence on the side of the road. This neighbor happened to be a vegetarian

and they got into quite a discussion on diet. The farmer simply could not understand how his vegetarian friend could possibly maintain enough energy to do any hard labor without meat and soon departed behind his plow sadly shaking his head. His vegetarian friend couldn't help but smile to himself as he departed thinking of the paradox—his farmer friend's horse was doing the hardest labor of all pulling the plow and the animal had never eaten meat in his whole life.

Heartbreaking stories are the norm when it comes to cancer. Wendy's story is another example of the point I'm trying to make in this chapter. When we met Wendy a lump had been found in her left breast. She had had a radical mastectomy. Eight months later, a lump appeared in her right breast and again a radical mastectomy was performed. Then they found cancer in the pelvic area and her ovaries were removed. Later they removed her adrenal glands. I guess Wendy and her husband finally decided that surgery was no longer the way to go because when the doctor wanted to operate again and take out the pituitary gland, her husband refused.

Wendy then started on an immunology program. While participating in this, she also went to Grapevine, Texas, and learned about Dr. Kelley's diet and started using some of his suggestions at the same time. Later, Wendy also went to Dr. Samchuck's clinic in Tecate, Mexico, where they use laetrile and at that time were giving much the same treatment as Dr. Contreras in Tijuana, Mexico, but again this was supplementary to the other two that she was already participating in. Incidentally, Dr. Samchuck is utilizing wheatgrass today.

She had several things going at one time and was afraid to give up any of them. I can understand her fear, I lived with it and it was a haunting, frightening, confusing merry-go-round. Many times I tried to encourage her to try the wheatgrass and the "living foods" diet. She was afraid to give up her other treatments, vitamins and high protein diet. In our research, we found that cancer people need to keep the protein on the low side because of a digestive problem. Prior to her death, she was back to eating pizzas and hamburgers again. My heart reached out to Wendy and her husband, knowing what they were going through but I was helpless. I couldn't convince them that since I had overcome cancer, that she could. I believe with all my heart that she could still be alive and as well as I am today.

For me to have Arn's encouraging support all the way with this has been just fantastic. He could have taken a cursory glance at Ann Wigmore's writings and decided that she was just another quack off on a tangent. I'm not sure that I could have done it if I had had to go it all alone. Not that the diet is that difficult but trying to go all the way with wheatgrass implants, the enemas, the colonic, the three weeks of digestive upsets in the beginning when my body was adjusting to the changeover to raw foods, etc. without his whole-hearted approval and moral support would have been very discouraging. Even now, to have to prepare two different meals three times a day would be difficult.

Another plus factor has been that we have been able to observe the response of his normal healthy body to the exact same "living foods" diet that is helping me. He feels better than he has ever felt in his life.

There are things that Arn can eat that I cannot as a "previous" cancer patient. Like dates. I got carried away one day and really got in trouble. I had brought home some gorgeous big organic dates. Dates are very high in natural sugar I didn't think much about it at the time, even though I knew by then that cancer patients simply cannot tolerate sugar or honey, it didn't register that the highly concentrated form of natural sugar in dates might give me a problem. I ate them with relish for a number of days without any visible problem, then whamo—I was suddenly back to that old tired feeling, and my lumps began to enlarge, and my hair got coarse again (I normally have very fine hair). That was the end of the dates for me. Right away I went and had a colonic irrigation (which I do about every three months anyway to keep the colon cleaned out) and went on a three day cleansing diet this time on citrus fruit, and in about a week's time I was back on my feet again.

When we elected to continue on this "living foods" diet strictly, we were cautioned by some doctors and nutritionists that we would be running the risk of becoming anemic besides having other problems arise from the fact that we were not eating enough protein or getting enough Vitamin B_{12}. We have stayed on the diet for over two and one half years now without any visible problems, and our feelings are probably best described by the word "euphoria." We never have any digestive upsets or colds, no need to take vitamins or food supplements, and we continue to feel great.

I have continued with the wheatgrass cocktails as well as the "living foods."

Any physical checkups that I have had with regular medical doctors have shown that I am in ideal condition, and according to the doctor, if I was measuring myself against an ideal chart, my physical condition in regard to blood and protein content and so forth is relatively perfect.

Out of our practical experience, it appears as though the doctor's and the nutritionist's concern is unfounded; that we *have* been receiving enough protein and blood building elements from the vegetables, fruits, nuts, sprouts, and wheatgrass that we have been eating. I believe that if the diet is not adhered to all the way, then it is possible the body would not absorb proteins. Also, taken in improper combinations, we believe that they would not be assimilated properly. But taken as we have learned to take them, we have found that these foods produce the proper protein for a very healthy and active person.

Have you heard the story of the sea gulls and the fishery at St. Augustine, Florida? In the business of catching, packing, and selling fish, the fishery threw all the scraps that were left, after cleaning the fish, directly into the ocean. For the sea gulls, it was like their meals were provided at no cost. The fishery was there for many years. The sea gulls came to depend upon the fishery. One day the fishery closed down. The sea gulls were left high and dry. They no longer knew how to scavenge in the ocean for their food. The oldest ones had forgotten how and the largest part of the sea gull population had never known anything but diving for the scraps from the fishery. They starved. In a very short time the sea gull population in that area was almost extinct.

Perhaps there is deeper wisdom than appears on the surface to that saying, "He who does not work shall not eat."

Most of us at one time or another have broken a bone and been put in a cast until the bone mended. That particular area of our body that was made immobile didn't have to do any work any longer. Do you remember when the cast came off? You had to teach it how to work all over. It took awhile before it was working at full capacity again.

Do you think it is possible that most bodies have forgotten how to process proteins from vegetables, fruits, nuts and sprouts simply because they have not had to do the work for so long? Could it be that our bodies have come to depend upon being supplied directly with protein?

If this is true, we believe that we have proven one

thing to ourselves. Being willing to experiment with our own bodies on this "living foods" diet, our bodies have re-learned in a natural way what they had forgotten because they didn't *have* to work for such a long time.

Ann Wigmore believes that in teaching good nutrition she is performing her God-given task in life. She believes that in showing others how to build their bodies (their temples in bible language) with life giving substances in place of dead foods or wrong foods, that only clog and create toxins thus poisoning the system leaving them open for all kinds of diseases, she can help to build a better world. She thinks that as more people learn how to set their bodies free by using only "living foods" to generate health and well-being, they will in turn tell others which will also help build a better world.

I realize that not everyone has what I would call a scientific mind. By this I mean a mind that is able to throw out all previous theories and hypotheses which do not square with the whole truth.

The whole truth of what I have been telling you in this book is that I am not only alive and well, but I have cancer under complete control by the use of the "living foods" diet which includes the use of wheatgrass juice.

My experience has been that if I deviate from this diet, the cancer cells return and multiply again.

Whether the whole truth comes out of a glass test tube or the test tube of practical experience is not important to me. What is important to me is whether it works or not.

The wheatgrass therapy and the "living foods" diet is working for me.

A SCIENTIST LOOKS AT ANN'S WHEATGRASS

Years ago Ann Wigmore experienced miraculous results after months of patient testing of the wheatgrass juice on her own shattered health. Where before she had been unable to work but for a few hours a day because of exhaustion and nervousness, the wheatgrass seemed to bring new alertness and energy into her body. Nothing seemed to be too difficult to accomplish, and work became a pleasure instead of a chore. Some of her friends tried it out with the same kind of results. She tells how she wasn't satisfied with this alone.

"I wanted an evaluation of the worth of wheatgrass chlorophyll from a scientist, one who had studied such things for many years and who had made a name for himself.

"Probably the foremost soil expert in the world, at the time, was Dr. G.H. Earp-Thomas of New Jersey. For more than half a century, his investigations had been aiding agriculturists all over the world to do their share in keeping up with the food needs of the earth's expanding population. I had known him slightly for a time and when I appeared in his laboratory and told him my story I found him most sympathetic. It was the first of many visits to his office and the beginning of an exciting adventure into realms I never realized existed. Dr. Earp-Thomas isolated over one hundred elements from fresh wheatgrass and concluded that it is a complete food.

"Now came more experiments. I separated six day old chicks into two groups of three chicks each. Each group was fed the best accepted type of chick food. But in one cage I mixed chopped up, freshly gathered wheatgrass with the food and placed a sprig of wheatgrass in the drinking water. At the end of a few weeks, all the chicks were healthy, but those receiving the wheatgrass had grown twice as large as the others. They were more alert and had feathered out better. Groups of rabbits and kittens, fed in similar fashion, showed the same results in size, weight and mentality.

I knew, then, that I had been entrusted with a precious secret to help people. Over the years, I have worked fervently to make this secret known. Now others are experimenting and discovering the wondrous benefits of wheatgrass.

"Years of experience have proven conclusively that the wheatgrass therapy is fundamentally correct. It follows the teaching of Hippocrates, the father of medicine who wisely said some twenty four hundred years ago, 'Let food be thy medicine.' Wheatgrass is not a 'cure' for anything. However, through scientific investigation and experimentation we know that it apparently furnishes the body with vital nourishment, which when missing seems to cause sickness and disease.

"Many physicians here in Boston have tested the miraculous effectiveness of the wheatgrass therapy. They have proven to their own satisfaction, that wheatgrass chlorophyll is definitely a new age food-medicine capable of solving the difficult problems of sick humanity.

"Since scores of physicians are certain that taking reasonable amounts of wheatgrass juice will not complicate any existing ailment, it seems just plain common sense that you test its miraculous possibilities upon your own body." [1]

WHEATGRASS THERAPY AND THE "LIVING FOODS" DIET

Changing eating habits requires a strong determination and there must be no underestimating the power of habits. My mind had to be willing to accept any change that I deemed necessary, and my movitation had to be strong. It is a narrow path that I had to walk to win over cancer. To this day, if I deviate from this narrow path, like the day I brought home those gorgeous, big, organically grown dates (See page 144), I can have a very real setback. With me, it was a matter of life or death. I had the will to live. It wasn't easy and I don't in any way mean to imply that it was, but as a consequence, the "living foods" diet has now become a real adventure.

On this "living foods" diet, sometimes a person's body takes awhile to adjust to the changes in eating. For the first few days, one may suffer headaches, nausea, fever, gas, or cramps, just depending upon how their particular body reacts to the change over to one hundred percent raw foods. Everybody is different. Plenty of rest is vital during this period to give the body a chance to clean itself of toxins stored away in cells or in fatty tissue, the accumulations of a lifetime of wrong foods, medications, or other abuses of the body.

As for myself, it took me three weeks to adjust to it. I had a lot of digestive problems, a lot of discomfort and a lot of gas. Once my body was conditioned to it, there was no problem. Prior to knowing that I had cancer, I used to have a lot of digestive problems which is characteristic of cancer. They have all disappeared, I just don't have *any* anymore.

MY FIRST THREE-DAY CLEANSING DIET

1. A three-day liquid cleansing diet was recommended to rid the body of toxic material before starting the regular diet regime (see Chapter Four, pages 70 & 72).
2. A colonic irrigation was strongly recommended before starting the three-day cleansing diet, (See

Chapter Four, pages 70 & 71) or at least sometime during the first three days. By checking the yellow pages of the phone book, I found a professional who gives colonics.

3. I alternated drinking Rejuvelac and the fruit juice I chose, every two hours, as much as I wanted, beginning with the Rejuvelac upon rising every morning. Rejuvelac is a drink made from wheat soaked in water overnight, rich in enzymes, minerals and vitamins. (See pages 153 & 154 for the recipe.) Fruit juice should be freshly juiced and strained (I used a juice extractor). I drank watermelon juice because it was in season (juiced whole including the rind). When watermelon is not available, other people have used citrus juice using a mixture of 12-14 oranges, 1-2 grapefruit, 1 lemon or lime. This was prepared and drunk throughout the day. No water was drunk. However, additional Rejuvelac could have been drunk less than an hour before or after juice.

4. I took two wheatgrass implants each day. The first enema and the first implant around 9:30 A.M. Two hours later, I took the second implant. (If it was inconvenient to take a second implant two hours later, I took another enema before the second implant.) Wheatgrass implants are taken to accelerate the cleansing and rejuvenating process. Certain people are not able to drink as much wheatgrass juice as they need at first. Their bodies are perhaps too toxic to handle adequate amounts.

By taking the wheatgrass implant the chlorophyll and the abscisic acid is absorbed directly into the system and much larger amounts may be handled by the body, resulting in quicker building and cleansing. (See pages 155 & 156 for my procedure for giving myself the wheatgrass implants.)

MY FIRST THREE DAY SCHEDULE

7:00 A.M.	2 oz. wheatgrass juice and a glass of Rejuvelac
7:30	Light exercise
9:00	Raw fruit juice, as much as I wanted
9:30	Enema and wheatgrass implant
11:00	2 oz. wheatgrass juice and a glass of Rejuvelac
11:30	Wheatgrass implant
1:00 P.M.	Raw fruit juice, as much as I wanted
3:00	2 oz. wheatgrass juice and a glass of Rejuvelac
5:00	Raw fruit juice, as much as I wanted
7:00	2 oz. wheatgrass juice and a glass of Rejuvelac
9:00 P.M.	Retire

HOW TO MAKE REJUVELAC

1 cup soft spring wheat, 3 cups of water.

Soak for twenty-four hours, then pour off the water into another container. Add three more cups to the same wheat for the next morning. Repeat from three to six days. Then start with fresh wheat again. (See page 205 for uses of this soaked wheat which is left from making Rejuvelac.) Drink a quart or more each day. This is a superior fermented drink filled with enzymes. Many researchers are now convinced that diseases are traceable to missing enzymes. Food that is fermented is filled with enzymes. Ann Wigmore shared a paper with us in which Dr. Kuhl, a German researcher had this to say regarding fermented foods, "The natural lactic acid and fermentive enzymes which are produced during the fermentation process, have a beneficial effect on the metabolism and a curative effect on disease. Lactic acid destroys harmful intestinal bacteria and contributes to the better digestion and assimilation of the nutrients. Fermented foods can be considered pre-digested foods. They are easily digested and assimilated even by persons with weak digestive organs. Fermented foods improve the intestinal tract and provide a proper environment for the body's own vitamin production within the intestines. They also help a person with constipation problems."

Ann also shared a letter she received from Dr. Harvey C. Lisle, a graduate in Chemical Engineering from the University of Ohio, with 15 years industrial experience in food testing laboratories, including both animal and human foods. He said that he made the

Rejuvelac as she suggested, using a ratio of two to one, water to wheat. Each day he poured off the Rejuvelac and ran a series of tests on it, one of them being a bacteria culture and found it to be loaded with lactobacilli and yeasts. He recommended that the fermenting wheat seeds in water be kept at a temperature of between 68 and 77 degrees for most desirable enzyme action.

Further comments that he made are, "The Rejuvelac is undoubtedly rich in proteins, carbohydrates, dextrines, saccharines, phosphates lactobacilli, saccharomyces and aspergillus oryzae. Amylases are derived from aspergillus oryzae and they have the faculty of breaking down large molecules of glucose, starch and glycogens. That is the reason the Rejuvelac is so beneficial to your digestion. Rejuvelac is related to beer although there is no alcoholic content. It is rich in the B vitamins. It is related to Brewers' Yeast and is high in protein. I might add that the 3 day Rejuvelac was superior to the 4th, 5th, 6th, and 7th day."

MY WHEATGRASS IMPLANTS

1. I purchased a good enema bag at a drugstore.
2. I found a place to purchase an eighteen inch catheter tube with glass connecting link. I removed the plastic nozzle from the enema bag and inserted the glass tube, then attached the catheter tube.

3. I had to take a warm water enema one half hour before each implant. If I was able to take my second implant within two hours of the first, I could eliminate the enema the second time.
4. One of the best and easiest positions for me to use for the enema was to lie on my left side, apply KY jelly lubrication to the catheter and insert the catheter partially or completely, releasing a small amount of water at a time. As a precautionary measure I allowed a small amount of water first to dribble through the tube. This expelled any air in the tube that might have caused discomfort. When there was a sense of fullness, I turned over to the right side and finished. If the first enema did not clean me out to a sufficient degree, I took another before beginning the implant.
5. I waited about a half hour after the enema before commencing the implant. After juicing the wheatgrass, I used it immediately. For my first implant I began with a third of a cup of wheatgrass chlorophyll juice undiluted, gradually increasing to a cup over the first three days. I proceeded with the implant as with an ordinary enema, but I retained the wheatgrass juice for twenty minutes, or longer but no longer than thirty minutes, or dissolved waste materials could have been reabsorbed into my blood stream. If I was having trouble holding the implant, I elevated the lower half of my body and pressed the rectum hard. I persisted, no matter how difficult it seemed at first, until I succeeded in accomplishing this feat.

Ann Wigmore teaches that implants of wheatgrass chlorophyll constitute the most effective blood cleanser and builder known; that chlorophyll implants cleanse the colon and can actually sustain human life when oral nourishment is impossible.

The chlorophyll molecule bears a striking resemblance to hemoglobin, the red pigment in human blood. The red blood pigment, a web of carbon, hydrogen, oxygen and nitrogen atoms grouped around a single atom of iron, is similar in every way to nature's green pigment except that its centerpiece is a single atom of magnesium. According to Adele Davis in her book, "Let's Eat Right to Keep Fit," magnesium is necessary to the action of some thirty enzymes in the body and that the best source is green leaves.

Lois Mattox Miller reported in an article on "Chlorophyll" in the Science News Letter:

"For ages men have puzzled over the question— 'What makes grass green?' About a century ago chemists segregated the green pigment in growing plants and named it chlorophyll, but until 1913 all attempts to explore the chlorophyll molecule failed. Then a German chemist, Dr. Richard Willstatter, made uncannily correct deductions about it. He likewise pointed out that the green miracle of nature is a process closely linked to the secret of life itself.

"A ray of sunlight strikes the green leaf and instantly the miracle is wrought. Within the plant, molecules of water and carbon dioxide are torn apart—a feat which the chemist can accomplish only with great difficulty and expense. First, there are only lifeless gas and water; then presto! these elements are transformed into living tissue and useful energy. Oxygen is released from the plant to revitalize the air we breathe. Units of energy, in natural sugars and other carbohydrates, are speedily manufactured and stored up in the living plant.

"All life energy comes from the sun. Green plants alone possess the secret of how to capture this solar energy, and pass it on to man and beast."

Most people think that adult bodies are built once. This is far from true, because our bodies are composed of individual cells like the bricks of a building, each cell having its own life and death. These cells are constantly wearing out, dying and being replaced by new cells, utilizing mostly new material taken in from our food. Nature has given us the glorious ability to rebuild ourselves day by day from the food we eat.

HOW I GROW WHEATGRASS

Every day at least ten trays of wheatgrass were brought to the kitchen at Ann Wigmore's mansion to be cut. There were at least one hundred trays in different stages of growth at all times.

The main planting rooms were in the basement of the mansion. Every bit of light from every window in the basement was well utilized for growing wheatgrass. Wheatgrass does not need full sun in order to grow well, just a little morning sun and a little afternoon sun, or one or the other. It starts best of all in complete darkness.

We had one full class session on growing wheatgrass, which I will expound upon as it is one of the more important elements in rejuvenating the life forces within the body. (Approximately seven months later, we were told that it was the abscisic acid in the wheatgrass that actually reversed the growth of tumors.)

The trays were 18 x 24 x 1 inches. Wet peat moss about a half inch thick is placed in the bottom. On top of this, the soil is put in loosely filling the tray (the soil should have earthworms in it). The dirt is then leveled off and smoothed over. All the way around the outside of the tray a small trench is channeled, giving the appearance of an upside down cake. This is to allow free movement of the water so that it does not sour the soil. The soil is then dampened, not saturated, with the water that the wheat seeds have been soaking in for twelve hours (seeds just barely covered). The soaked wheat seeds are placed on top, one kernel touching another in an even layer like icing a cake, and gently patted down. (Do not allow any kernels to fall in the trench or they will rot and become rancid and ruin the whole tray.) The layer of wheat seed is covered with six to eight pages of soaked newspaper (black and white section only—no color). Lay them very carefully on top of the seed, then wrap the whole tray, paper and all, with thin black plastic. Tuck the plastic under the tray to prevent the moisture from escaping. Place in a dark area to sprout.

In approximately two days if it is warm, or three days if it is cooler, the plastic will begin to rise and droplets of water will form on the underside of the plastic. The wheat sprouts push the newspaper up right along with the plastic. Now the newspaper and the plastic are removed. The wheat sprouts will be white and about one half to three quarters of an inch high. These are now ready to be placed in a window where they need to be watered once a day with a sprinkling can. Do not saturate, just dampen, just a hint of moisture in the bottom of the trench.

When the grass is about seven or eight inches high, it is ready for the first cutting. It is then allowed to grow back for a second cutting, just as a farmer gets two cuttings.

Grown in this manner, wheatgrass can be grown indoors in apartments or houses. No holes are in the bottom of the pans so the trays will not hurt any surface where they are placed. This is another reason why the watering is so carefully regulated.

We also learned how to recycle the soil. As the trays are harvested, they are turned upside down, removing the soil and the roots which remain matted together from the tray. These mats are placed in a dark area of the basement. Pulp is taken from the juicing that is done in the kitchen and placed between these one inch thick mats. When the mats are stacked about four feet high and four or five trays in length, they are covered with black plastic and left for approximately three months. The worms work in and out and eat up the root system and the juice pulp, leaving a richer soil ready to be used again. (The ecologists and the conservationists should go wild over this one.)

Grown in a greenhouse, it is a little less complicated. Holes can be punched in the bottoms of the trays. There would be no need for the trenches as the water would have proper drainage through these holes. The harvested mats could be buried in the ground while the worms break down the root system.

For apartment living, the soil can be recycled right in a garbage can. Anyone can garden indoors with a little ingenuity.

MY "LIVING FOODS" DIET

After the liquid diet, I broke it with a mild fruit, then some sprouts and greens, nothing heavy. I followed the rules for thorough chewing of my food for good digestion. I eat all my foods raw, and get them organically grown whenever possible. I chew all raw vegetables and fruit carefully, preferably until they are virtually a liquid, even the grated raw vegetables. If they are finely chopped or grated, I eat them right away, or twenty to twenty-five percent of the vitamins would be lost. I disciplined myself to smaller amounts in the beginning.

MY ORIGINAL SCHEDULE

7:00 A.M.   8 oz. Rejuvelac (now, I mostly get it in sauces)

7:30	Light exercise
8:00	*Breakfast*—In summer I usually eat melons, sometimes half a watermelon, sometimes a whole canteloupe, honey-dew, crenshaw etc. In winter, I usually have citrus fruit. Arn also mixes soaked wheat and millet for a breakfast cereal. I seem to do better without this extra protein.
9:00	Enema and implant for two more weeks after I returned home.
10:00	8 oz. of the Green Cocktail, 20 raw almonds (see page 181 for recipe)
11:00	Implant for two more weeks after I returned home.
12:00 noon	*Lunch*—Tossed green meal salad, (see pages 195-203 for recipes), some raw vegetable sticks, and sandwiches (see page 192 for recipe).
4:00 P.M.	8 oz. of the Green Cocktail
6:00	*Dinner*—Fruit again in correct combinations (see recipes pages 182 & 183) Sometimes I have a cup of hot herb tea one half hour before eating, or two hours after eating. My favorite is Garden Treat.

After my energy had returned, and I was feeling pretty good consistently, I stopped the implants and continued to make progress with the wheatgrass cocktails and the "living foods" diet alone.

Other bonuses from the "living foods" diet (besides

conquering cancer) are:
1. My appetite is better than at any time before in my life.
2. The delicate food flavors are so much more noticeable and the food tastes positively delicious.
3. I can eat all I want without fear of gaining weight or getting fat. (I eat well!)
4. I never have to clean the oven or the stove! (I had a cover made for the stove and now keep my juicer on top.)

WHY SHOULD I SPROUT SEEDS?

Sprouts will grow in any climate, may be planted any day of the year, require no soil or sunshine, cause no waste in preparation and rival meat in nutritive value. They are full of vitamins, minerals, and quantities of protein in the purest form and are readily digested since they contain within themselves high quantities of enzymes.

Sprouts are an excellent source of Vitamins A, B-Complex, C, D, E, G, K, and even U, and minerals such as calcium, magnesium, phosphorous, chlorine, potassium, sodium, and silicon, all in natural forms which the body can readily assimilate. All sprouts contain vitamins A, B, and C equivalent to that found in fruit. Alfalfa sprouts are also rich in vitamins D, E, G, K, and U. [2]

We learned from Ann Wigmore that Dr. Paul Burnholder of Yale University measured the following *increases* in the B-complex vitamin content of dry oats after only *five days of sprouting*; (and the figures for Vitamin C show a similar pattern)

Biotin	50%
Folic Acid	600%
Inositol	100%
Niacin Acid	500%
Pantothenic Acid	200%
Pyrodoxine (B6)	500%
Riboflavin (B2)	1,350%
Thiamin (B1)	10%

Take a soybean, mung bean, alfalfa seed, or a wheat berry and soak it overnight. Keep it moist and rinsed and in a very short time, it will come to life. The seed will germinate, and a tiny sprout will poke its way out and begin to grow. This simple miraculous change is of the greatest nutritional significance. Research shows that the sprout in its first days of life is a veritable vitamin factory.

Dr. Clive M. McCay of Cornell University worked on the possibility of promoting sprouted soybeans as an all-around good nutritious food as far back as World War II when we in the United States were fearing further food shortages. In his published report, he says that soybean sprouts are rich in protein and fat, minerals, including calcium and usable iron and vitamins.[3]

We learned from Dr. Francis Pottenger, Jr. of Monrovia, California, that the sprouts develop into a complete protein capable of sustaining life. While you watch them sprout, protein is manufactured before your very eyes, along with vitamins.

Protein is constructed of twenty-two building blocks called amino acids, of which eight have been found essential in the food requirements of people. The other fourteen can be made by the cells from fat or sugar combined with the nitrogen freed from the breakdown of used proteins. From the eight essential amino acids, we can synthesize the others we require. All eight of these essential amino acids must be present together in a complete meal as they complement each other's qualities. If one of the eight is missing, then the remaining amino acids cannot be utilized and fail to provide in the way they were designed. These eight essential amino acids are: Leucine and Isoleucine, Lysine, Methionine, Phenylalanine, Tryptophane, Threonine, and Valine.

Proteins containing the eight essential amino acids in generous amounts are called complete or adequate. Many of the seeds contain complete proteins, one of the highest in value being the sunflower seed. Sprout the sunflower seed and it just gains in value. The value of any protein depends on the number and amount of essential amino acids it contains.

These so-called essential amino acids must be supplied in the diet if health is to be maintained; each of them is as important as is any vitamin.

The studying that I have done regarding sprouts has given me a great respect for their protein content as well as their vitamin content. (See the Recommended Reading List for books about sprouts.) Physiology teaches us that man lives by the process of converting some of his food into building blocks of protein which replace his cells as they wear out, and by burning other food as energy which enables him to play, work, and enjoy life. We all learned in school that the various substances of which food is made (carbohydrates, proteins, and fats) are "changed" by the digestive process and in this "change" they become useful to our bodies. Enzymes play a vital part in these "changes" which enable us to digest our food and use it for energy and for rebuilding cells. There are two circumstances that disturb the activity of enzymes, cold and heat. Cold inactivates them. Between 32 and 104 degrees Fahrenheit, enzymes are very active. But when you heat them to a point above 122 degrees Fahrenheit, enzymes are permanently destroyed.

We do know that enzymes are found in abundance in raw food. In cooked food, enzymes are non-existent, however, we do have organs within our bodies that produce enzymes. We wonder if it would not greatly benefit health, if those organs didn't have to work overtime supplying enzymes which should logically be supplied by food?

The intricacies of enzyme action are lengthy. Suffice it to say we know that there are enzymes in sprouts, because seeds cannot germinate without enzymes. (We eat all our sprouts raw, we do not cook any of our food.)

Not only do all these qualifications sound utopian, but sprouting can be great fun!

HOW TO SPROUT

Almost any seed, grain or legume, can be sprouted, although most devotees prefer alfalfa, soybeans, mung beans, lentils, peas, and the cereal grains— wheat, barley, oats, buckwheat and rye. Unhulled sesame and sunflower seeds, radish, mustard, red clover, fenugreek, corn, lima beans, pinto and kidney beans, chick peas and nearly any other seed can be sprouted successfully. It is wise to purchase organically grown seed to be sure that it has not been sprayed or chemically treated in any way.

1. Wash seeds thoroughly and pick out any chaff or cracked seeds.
2. Place three tablespoons of alfalfa or any of the smaller seeds, or half a cup of the larger seeds (mung beans, lentils, chick peas, sunflower seeds) into a two quart jar (preferably a wide mouth jar) and cover with screening (plastic or wire) or double thickness cheese cloth, securing with a rubber band or a canning ring, or even a clean worn-out nylon stocking.
3. Cover the seeds with water (room temperature) and let the seeds soak overnight. Alfalfa and the smaller seeds need only soak 3-4 hours.
4. Next morning, pour off the enriched, enzyme-

packed soak water and drink it or save to water your plants or your garden.

5. Place your containers, with seeds well drained, on its side, in a warm environment, where you can see them so you will remember to tend them. (If you don't like the clutter of seeing them, they sprout just as well or perhaps a little better inside a dark cupboard.) In the evening, rinse and drain the seeds again to keep them moist. During the next few days, be sure to keep the seeds moist by rinsing and draining them morning and night. In about three days you will see the tiny sprouts.

6. Actually sprouts are ready for use as soon as the sprout is seen, however, the longer they sprout, the more nourishment. Sprouts are more tender when young and are less delicious if *too* long. Most sources agree that:

   —Alfalfa sprouts are best when 1 to 2 inches long.
   —Wheat sprouts are most delicious when the sprout is the length of the seeds.
   —Soybean and pea sprouts are good short or long.
   —Mung bean sprouts are best when 1½ to 3 inches long.
   —Lentil sprouts, one inch.
   —Sunflower seed sprouts, when no longer than the seed.

7. They are at the peak of their vitamin potency 3 to 4 days after germination. If you have sprouted

your seeds in the dark and they are the desired length, expose them to light until they turn green. When the green appears, Vitamin A and chlorophyll has been manufactured.[4] Refrigerate them until they are used.

There is as much variety in the taste of sprouts as in the "traditional" vegetables, and no limit to the ways in which they can be used in menus to yield their nutritional treasure. Why don't you try them all?

NO-NO'S FOR EYDIE MAE, THE CANCER PATIENT

1. No sugar in any form—raw, brown, or white.
2. No honey—raw or pasteurized.
3. No salt (I use granulated kelp instead).
4. No dairy products in any form—milk, cream, cheese, yogurt, ice cream, eggs.
5. No fat—butter, margarine.
6. No dried fruits—(the dehydrating process converts this food into a highly concentrated form of sugar).
7. No meat, fish, or poultry.
8. No supplementary vitamins are needed or recommended because as soon as your body has gone through the cleansing process, the body converts the live food to all the vitamins required.
9. No white flour.
10. No coffee or tea (with the exception of herb teas).

11. No alcoholic beverages.
12. No liquids at mealtime as this dilutes the digestive enzymes—drink all liquids at least one half hour before meals or two hours after.
13. For myself, I prefer no protein after lunch. The cancer patient has a problem digesting proteins and it takes protein a long time to digest. I utilize fruit only for my evening meal. This enables me to sleep really great because fruits digest easier and faster than vegetables and proteins. I experimented on my own.

EASY DOES IT

1. I go easy on the oils as they coat the stomach wall and can hinder food assimilation. I use cold pressed vegetable oil base salad dressings, but I go very easy on them and do not use them regularly.
2. I go easy on the proteins as cancer patients have a protein digestive problem. Soy products are too high in protein for me. I experimented with the list of proteins given; it may be different for others. I do well with avocadoes, almonds, sunflower seeds, and sprouts.

SOME QUESTIONS PEOPLE ASK

What is the question you get asked the most?

When you don't eat any meat, how do you have enough energy to keep you going?

The truth is that I have more energy now than I have had in years.

Do you find that you get tired of eating salads?

No, we haven't. When checking through the long list of vegetables and fruits, it can easily be seen that there is more variety to choose from than if a choice had to be made from the different kinds of meat. Towards the end of winter, variety in fruit is scarce and we are are really glad when the spring fruits come in, but we have favorite vegetable dinner salads (use recipes in the back of the book) of which we never get tired.

If a person doesn't have cancer, can they use honey in the "living foods" diet?

Yes.

Does your husband, Arn, stick as strictly to the diet as you do?

No, sometimes when he is at a business luncheon and a raw salad is not available, he'll have a tuna fish salad sandwich, or another favorite, but not often. More often he plans his luncheons to occur where raw salads are available.

Do you buy your salad dressing or do you make your own?

Mostly I make my own, (I use a lot of lemon juice plain) but I do buy one faithfully. It's called "Lecinaise." It's made of cold pressed oils, lecithin, lemon juice and apple cider vinegar. There are no eggs in it and it tastes exactly like mayonnaise. I can't tell the difference.

Is it harmful to eat watermelon rind?
No, actually you can juice the whole watermelon, green and white rind as well as the red part.
Can brewers' yeast be used with the diet?
Yes.
Are there any fruits or vegetables that you cannot eat?
I eat all raw, fresh fruits and vegetables, but no dried fruits, and no canned fruits or vegetables. I also avoid too much onion simply because it doesn't agree with me.
Does your husband, Arn, drink the wheatgrass juice also?
Occasionally, not regularly. He has a strong, healthy body and puts only healthy foods into his body, getting plenty of chlorophyll from the leafy greens I put in our salads, and doesn't seem to need it. I think he drinks a "Green Cocktail" with me every now and then just to keep me company.
Do you use a special grinder for grinding seeds like sesame seeds?
Yes, I use a "coffee, seed and nut grinder" that I bought at a health food store, but many of the blenders do a good job on them also.
Do you know of any inexpensive juicer that juices wheatgrass?
Yes, I can recommend two: Chop Rite#27 Health Fountain, Chop Rite Manufacturing Company, Pottstown, Pa. 19464 (cost approx. $40.00) and Paul Electric Kitchen Machine, 6880 Tower, San Diego, Calif. 92115. 714-465-5285.

When you cut your vegetables up raw, do you peel them?

No, not usually as they are more nutritious with skins. Sometimes, for company, if I know they are very new to the idea of raw food meals, I'll peel them.

Doesn't watermelon give you a lot of gas?

Not when eaten alone or with other melons only. When it's using different enzymes to digest the other foods, the mixture of enzymes is what causes the gas.

What about shopping in a regular supermarket for your fruit and vegetables?

If you can get your fruit and vegetables organically grown, this is best, but not everybody has access to them. As a matter of necessity, supermarket fruit and vegetables may have to be used.

Are there restrictions on combining vegetables as there are on combining fruits?

No, you can combine any of the vegetables and be trouble free.

How do you juice wheatgrass?

I cut the wheatgrass off at the roots when it is seven inches high. Then I cut the grass in about two inch lengths before putting it in the juicer. Arn has put a motor on my juicer to make it an easier job. A regular meat grinder can be used, but it takes longer and usually requires straining through cheesecloth.

Do hot peppers bother your stomach?

No, hot peppers are very good for you, they have a lot of vitamin A and C in them. I have read of cases of colitis being cured with hot cayenne pepper which was put in gelatin capsules and eaten with every meal. It was a special African capsicum pepper. It has a healing effect. I have also heard of a study that was made in Texas near the Mexican border where the blood cholesterol was very low in the people. It turned out that it was due to the hot peppers they ate.

Is the wheatgrass juice the main key to getting rid of the cancer?

Yes, it is a must, but I believe the live foods has to go with it to maintain health.

If you go out to eat in a restaurant, what do you eat?

I simply order a good size raw salad and have them serve it without dressing, then add what dressing I want. Sometimes I ask for lemon to be served with it.

My husband has an enormous appetite, how would he ever be satisfied with a salad?

I didn't think that I could be satisfied with a salad, either, but I am, and now I prefer it to a steak; I'm not even tempted anymore. Remember, my life was immediately at stake; it makes a lot of difference. I decided that if it was going to be either a steak, or a hamburger, or a pizza, or *me*, the choice was easy, I chose me.

Is it really true that you can eat as much as you want and not gain weight?

Yes, at first we lost all excess weight. Then our bodies seemed to level off at our natural weight, and it stays right there. I can eat half a watermelon for breakfast, have carrot juice with my wheatgrass juice mid-morning, eat as much as my stomach will hold at lunch and again at supper and my weight remains between 104-107 consistently, no matter how much I eat. Arn leveled off at 132 and the same is true for him.

What is the Bible bread that you eat?

Bible bread is an unleavened bread made from one hundred percent whole wheat flour, no eggs, no sugar, no honey, just a little sea salt, nothing in it to raise the dough and no preservatives. This can be bought at a health food store.

Why isn't pineapple on the no-no list? Isn't it high in sugar content?

It's a different kind of natural sugar that the enzymes are able to handle. (Grapes, too.) It's not highly concentrated like in the dried fruits.

Are there any rules against sprinkling ground nuts or seeds over fruit?

Yes, this is a poor food combination and should be avoided. Nuts combine well with any vegetable, or protein, not fruit.

Is wheatgrass good for anything else besides killing cancer cells?

Some of the other almost unbelievable things that Dr. Earp-Thomas proved when he was experimenting with wheatgrass in his laboratory are:

1. That fruits and vegetables, contaminated by sprays, were cleaned thoroughly by a wisp of wheatgrass placed in the water in which they were washed.

2. That when utilizing the wheatgrass juice for the sterilization of his instruments and for washing his hands when working with various types of bacteria, he found it to be more

effective than boiling water.

3. That tests showed when he added a few blades of wheatgrass to fluoridated water for several minutes, no fluorine was traceable. Later, an official of the Water Department of New York City tested some fluoridated water in which a small bunch of wheatgrass had been swished. He could find no trace of fluorine.

Also, while we were at Ann Wigmore's Health Institute in Boston, we learned how as the body regains its health after being on the "living foods" diet, including the wheatgrass therapy, all kinds of problems that people have, clear up. Some of them mentioned were: arthritis, asthma, sinus problems, and allergies.

Since you have conquered your cancer, do you still have the lumps that appeared some time after your original lumpectomy?

Yes, I still have those small lumps, but they have reduced in size from the size of a walnut down to the size of a pea.

Are you free from any pain connected with your cancer?

Strangely, each time the lumps decrease a little more in size, I have pain in those areas (of an intensity of about #4). Arn and I developed a scale from one to ten indicating the intensity of the pain when I was enduring constant pain for quite a period before we went to Boston (#10 being the most painful).

Would you consider your use of the wheatgrass juice and "living foods" to conquer cancer a similar thing to the use of insulin to control diabetes?

There are no unpleasant side effects from the use of wheatgrass and "living foods" to conquer cancer (after the body adjusts to the change to completely raw foods). We have found that we just get more and more a feeling of well-being, whereas in the use insulin, I understand that there are many varied reactions and side effects to the different forms of insulin.

If you had it to do over, would you have had the lumpectomy?

No.

Did you have to go to Ann Wigmore's to go on the "Living Foods" Diet?

No. However, I'm glad that I did as my meals were prepared for me as I was getting used to the diet and learning how to prepare the food. My enthusiasm was higher eating with other people in the same manner. It was easier for me to learn "how" when others were demonstrating for me. I could start immediately with the wheatgrass therapy, whereas it takes me about a week to ten days to grow wheatgrass. It made everything easier for me.

Where can I get the wheat berries?

Most health food stores usually have both the hard, red winter wheat and the soft, spring wheat (for Rejuvelac) in stock or can order it for you. Remember, fumigated wheat will not sprout.

8 | RECIPES

WHEATGRASS COCKTAIL

First day

1 T. wheatgrass chloro-
phyll juice
4oz. Rejuvelac
Mix together and drink.

After the second day—
increase gradually to:
2 oz. wheatgrass chloro-
phyll juice
6 oz. Rejuvelac
Mix together and drink.

THE GREEN COCKTAIL

1 qt. of carrot juice
1 stalk of celery juiced
1 fresh tomato

8 oz. of wheatgrass juice
Several sprigs of parsley
Kelp to taste

Blend together all ingredients in your blender. Drink some immediately and the rest spread out over a few hours.

Wheatgrass is not compatible with fruits. Wait one hour after fruit or fruit juice is taken before taking wheatgrass juice. All meals other than fruit may be taken immediately or shortly after your wheatgrass cocktail. Never take wheatgrass juice right after a meal.

FOOD COMBINATIONS—FRUIT

Because of the different enzymes needed to digest the different fruits, there are certain rules to follow as to what fruits combine well together for one meal. All fruits listed in one classification (in one box) may be combined and eaten with one another, but *not* with any other classification of fruit. (Ex. Melons should be eaten alone.) Do not mix fruits with vegetables.

Acid Fruits

Orange	Lemon	Sour Peach
Grapefruit	Lime	Sour Plum
Pineapple	Sour Apple	Tangelo
Pomegranate	Sour Grape	Tangerine

Sub-Acid Fruits

Fresh Fig	Sweet Peach	Huckleberry
Pear	Sweet Apple	Mango
Sweet Cherry	Apricot	
Papaya	Sweet Plum	

Sweet Fruits

Bananas
Grapes (sweet)
Fresh Figs (sweet)
Cherries (sweet)

Persimmons
Mangos
Papayas

Sub-Sweet Fruits

Plums
Apricots
Cherries (tart)

Nectarines
Peaches (sweet)
Grapes (tart)

Melons

Watermelon
Cantaloupe
Muskmelon
Honey Dew

Crenshaw
Persian
Casaba

Berries

Blueberries
Strawberries
Boysenberries

Raspberries
Blackberries

BONANZA SPLIT

2 bananas, sliced in half
  lengthwise
1 papaya, cut up in
  pieces
1 mango, cut up

2 bunches seedless grapes
1 persimmon, diced fine
2 banana split dishes

Place the bananas lengthwise in the bottom of the banana split dishes. Put a pile of grapes in the center on top of the banana. Pile up papaya pieces on one end and mango pieces on the other end on top of the banana. Sprinkle persimmon on top.

APRICOT DELIGHT

6 apricots, pitted and
  sliced
2 sweet apples cut up

Huckleberries
1 pear diced
2 green plates

Mix together sliced apricots, cut up apples, and huckleberries. Arrange on green plates (if you have them). Sprinkle with diced pear.

SPLENDID TRIO

4 fresh figs
1 papaya, sliced length-
  wise peeled)

Bing cherries
2 clear glass or white
  salad plates

Arrange the fruit in three sections on the plates, piling the Bing cherries high.

PINEAPPLE SPECIAL

1 cup fresh pineapple cut up (and two round slices)
½ cup cut up orange

1 sour apple cut up
1 pomegranate

Mix together cut up pineapple, orange and sour apple. Arrange on top of a full round slice of fresh pineapple. Sprinkle pomegranate seeds on top.

UNCOOKED APPLESAUCE

3 organic sweet apples
½ cup water

Cut up the apples, peels, cores, seeds and all. Pour ½ cup water into blender. Drop in the cut up apples. Do not blend too long, or they will oxidize. Eat right away. If your apples are not organically grown, remove the pits and do not use.

PINEAPPLE GRAPEFRUIT JUICE

1 fresh pineapple
1 fresh grapefruit

Put the pineapple through a juice extractor, core and all. Add to this the juice of 1 fresh grapefruit and shake. Served chilled, or with crushed ice, it makes a nice party drink.

BAHAMA DELIGHT

1 coconut

Prepare the coconut as described on page 74. Enjoy the fresh coconut milk. Break the flesh of the coconut into small pieces, grind to a powder and place in blender with small amount of water, or cut up into small pieces and gradually add to water while blender is in motion. Blend until it is changed into a milk-like liquid.

TROPICAL SPECIAL

1 banana   ½ cup water
1 papaya, cut up

Pour water in blender. Add banana and papaya while blender is in motion. Blend until smooth. Add more water if needed for desired consistency. Serve in clear glasses or bowls. Makes a delicious enzyme filled drink.

A mango added to the Tropical Special is also delicious.

FOOD COMBINATIONS—VEGETABLES AND PROTEINS

All vegetables may be combined and eaten with any of the listed protein foods, or with one another, but not with fruit. One exception to the rule: Pineapple may be combined with leafy greens and wheatgrass, eaten alone, or combined with sweet fruits.

VEGETABLES

Artichokes	Dandelion
Asparagus	Egg Plant
Avocados	Endive
Bamboo Sprouts	Escarole
Banana Squash	Garlic
Beets and Tops	Green Beans
Broccoli	Hubbard Squash
Brussel Sprouts	Jicama
Cabbage	Kale
Cardoon	Leeks
Carrots	Lettuce
Cauliflower	Mustard
Celery	Mushrooms
Chicory	Okra
Chinese Cabbage	Onions
Chives	Parsley
Collards	Parsnips
Corn	Peas
Cucumber	Pea pods (young)

Peppers, Hot
Peppers, Sweet
Potatoes
Pumpkin
Radish
Rhubarb
Rutabagas
Scallions (green onions)
Soy Bean Sprouts

Spinach
Summer Squash
Sweet Potatoes
Swiss Chard
Tomato
Turnip
Water Cress
Yams
Zucchini

PROTEINS

raw unsalted nuts
(except peanuts)
cereal grains
avocados
seeds, (sunflower, sesame,
pumpkin, etc.)
soy beans and dry beans

sprouts (alfalfa, wheat,
lentils, soy bean, mung
bean, rye, oats, etc.)
coconuts

GAZPACHO
A Chilled Mexican Soup—GOOD!

fresh tomatoes
1 large cucumber
1 large onion, peeled
or green onions
1 bell pepper
1 can pimiento

¼ cup olive oil (cold pressed)
¼ cup vinegar (apple cider)
1 chili pepper (I like the
Floral Gem)
kelp
garlic (chopped fine)
vegetable seasoning
1 can sliced ripe olives

Put tomatoes in blender and puree to make about 18-20 ounces. Cut cucumber, onion and pepper into cubes. Put in blender. Add pimiento, kelp, garlic seasoning, oil and vinegar. Puree. Chill at least 3 hours. Also chill 6 serving bowls and a soup tureen.

Chop fresh tomato, cucumber, onion, green pepper. Place in separate bowls. Chill olives in small bowl. Sprinkle over top of each serving.

VEGETABLE SOUP

3 carrots grated
2 cups fresh peas
several stalks of celery

2 T. olive oil
Rejuvelac or water
kelp and vegetable
    seasoning

Blend in blender and season with kelp and vegetable seasoning to taste. Add Rejuvelac or water to the desired soup consistency. Top with sprouts if desired.

CUCUMBER SOUP

1 cucumber
1 zucchini
1 small avocado

1 cup Rejuvelac
fresh lime juice to taste
Vegetable seasoning and
    garlic to taste

Blend all ingredients together to a soup consistency. Good on a hot day.

BUFFET SOUP

vegetable seasoning
hot water
sesame sauce
chopped tomato

grated carrots
grated onions
favorite sprouts
bits of cucumber

Blend vegetable seasoning, hot water and sesame sauce. Add vegetables to broth and serve. Or serve vegetables in separate bowls and let each person select the vegetables to add to his individual bowl of broth. Garnish with bits of cucumber.

UNCOOKED CORN CHOWDER

2 tomatoes
fresh corn on the cob
   (uncooked)
1 cup of water

¼ cup sunflower seed
   sprouts (sprouted only as
   long as the seed)
¼ cup chopped celery

Peel tomatoes and mash. Cut corn off the cob. Have the celery ready. Heat the water to no more than 120 degrees. Take the water off the stove and add the vegetables. If desired season with vegetable seasoning. Enzymes are killed above 120 degrees. If you prefer, you can serve this cold as well. (A candy thermometer works well for determining the heat of the water.)
   Sprinkle rye sprouts into soup just before serving. They add a mouthwatering tang.

TOMATO VEGETABLE SOUP

1½ cups freshly chopped
   tomatoes
3 cups finely chopped
   celery
3 cups grated carrots

1 cup parsley chopped fine
   (save 2 T.)
¼ cup green onion, chopped
   fine
1 tsp. kelp

Blend all ingredients except 2 T. parsley to sprinkle on top with sprouts if desired. Add Rejuvelac or water to soup for desired consistency. (This makes a delicious vegetable juice by adding another quart of water and straining.)

LENTIL SOUP

1 cup slightly sprouted
   lentils
1 large onion
2 cups water
1 medium uncooked
   potato diced
½ tsp. sweet basil

½ cup chopped celery
½ cup parsley
½ tsp. vegetable oil (or soy)
kelp and vegetable seasoning to taste

Blend together water, lentil sprouts, onions, celery, parsley, oil and sweet basil. Top with diced potato, kelp, and vegetable seasoning to taste.
Use lots of parsley! Sprinkle it in your soups. Toss it in your salads. Cancer doesn't like to grow in a potassium base and parsley has lots of potassium in it.

EYDIE MAE'S CALIFORNIA SANDWICH

Bible bread (buy at
  Health Food Store)
avocado—sliced or
  mashed
kelp and vegetable
  seasoning
lemon juice
lecinaise

raw mushrooms
hot chili peppers, chop-
  ped fine
sweet bell peppers, chopped
  fine
sunflower seeds
alfalfa sprouts

Mash your avocado or slice and season with kelp, vegetable seasoning and lemon juice. Warm your bread, split your loaf and spread each side with lecinaise (an eggless mayonnaise). Spread with mashed or sliced avocado. Add hot chili peppers or sweet bell peppers depending upon your taste, or both. Add raw mushroom slices and sprinkle with sunflower seeds. Top with alfalfa sprouts (a good covering). I serve them open face at home, but put the second half of the loaf on top for a box lunch (or a brown bag). Delicious!

EYDIE MAE'S CALIFORNIA TOSTADA
for special occasions only (or guests) due to cooked pinto beans.

corn tortillas (without
  preservatives)
warm cooked pinto beans

tossed green salad

avocado dip
alfalfa sprouts or mung
  bean sprouts
radishes, parsley and
  cherry tomatoes

Blend pinto beans in a little hot water (or mash).
Spread on tortilla (heated). Add a layer of tossed salad.
Top this with avocado dip. Top this with sprouts.
Garnish with radishes, parsley and cherry tomatoes.
Serve open face with garnishes on the side.

NUT LOAF
(FILLING FOR SANDWICH OR SIDE DISH)

1 cup carrots
½ cup chopped parsley
1 clove garlic (optional)
ground nuts

1 cup tomatoes
½ cup bell pepper pieces
2 T. oil
Your favorite herb (mine
is sage or dill)

Put all through a food grinder, mix and pack into a
loaf pan to serve or make sandwich.

GARDEN TACOS

corn tortillas

avocados, sliced
pinto bean sprouts
   mashed
sunflower seeds
vegetarian cheese (non-
   dairy)
raw mushrooms sliced

Anaheim peppers (mildly
   hot) chopped fine
Floral Gem peppers (hot)
   chopped fine
alfalfa sprouts or other
   favorite sprouts
cherry tomatoes, halved,
   or sliced tomatoes
red salsa sauce
green tomatillo sauce

Combinations are endless. Start with corn tortillas (first wrapped in foil and heated in your oven), sliced avocados, or pinto bean sprouts mashed, or vegetarian cheese, and build from there with your favorite sprouts, topping with either red salsa sauce, or the green tomatillo sauce, sunflower seeds, tomatoes, and chopped peppers. Make your own Dagwood.

RED SALSA TACO SAUCE

2 cups fresh tomatoes blended
1 can (small) peeled green ortega chilis or 2 fresh minced and seeded
1 sweet onion chopped fine

2 cloves garlic, crushed through garlic press
Juice of 2 lemons
1 very ripe avocado diced finely
1 T. kelp

Mix all together and refrigerate at least 24 hours.

GREEN TOMATILLO TACO SAUCE

1 cup finely chopped tomatillos (Mexican tart green tomatoes)
½ cup finely chopped onion or 5 or 6 green onions chopped

2-3 T. chopped hot chili peppers
1 T. Kelp
pinch of fresh chopped coriandrum (chinese parsley or mexican cilatro)

Mix together and refrigerate at least 2 hours. Makes 1½ cup.

TOSSED SALAD

romaine lettuce
red leaf lettuce
head lettuce
beet tops
sliced tomatoes
thinly sliced cauliflower

thinly sliced cabbage (red)
chopped bell pepper
alfalfa sprouts
sunflower seed sprouts
raw grated beets
herb dressing

Add any small pieces of raw vegetables left over from previous meals and toss with Herb dressing. Garnish with sliced radishes and raw mushrooms. Use any of your favorite vegetables as substitutes or additions.

ARMENIAN SALAD

4 large tomatoes peeled
   and cubed
2 cucumbers, diced
2 stalks celery sliced
½ cup finely chopped
   onion (red)
½ bunch watercress,
   chopped

¼ cup chopped parsley
pinch of basil, dried mint,
   or 1 tsp. fresh mint
¼ cup lemon juice
2 T. cold pressed oil
2 tsp. vegetable seasoning
ground kelp to taste

Combine tomatoes, cucumbers, celery, onion, watercress, parsley, basil and mint, then toss. Sprinkle with lemon juice, oil, vegetable seasoning and kelp, then toss again. Many times we use just lemon juice, kelp and vegetable seasoning without oil.

LEMON HERB DRESSING

1 stalk celery and leaves
1 small green onion and
  tops chopped very fine
1 tsp. vegetable broth and
  seasoning
½ tsp. sea salt (or 1 tsp.
  kelp)

2 sprigs parsley
¼ tsp. dried sweet basil
⅔ cup cold pressed salad
  oil
1/16 tsp. marjoram
juice of one lemon

Shake vigorously in covered jar till blended. Allow to stand in refrigerator till flavors are blended.

SPINACH, MUSHROOM AND RED ONION SALAD

½ lb. mushrooms, sliced
3 T. lemon juice
⅓ cup safflower oil
  (cold pressed)
1 red onion sliced and
  separated

2 cups torn spinach leaves
5 cups torn salad greens
  (red, romaine, or other)
vegetable seasoning and
  kelp to taste

Marinate mushrooms in combined lemon juice and oil. Toss with onion, spinach and greens, then season with vegetable seasoning and kelp.

ANN WIGMORE'S "COMPLETE MEAL SALAD"

The "Complete Meal Salad" contains full protein in quantity and quality, all eight of the essential amino acids, a total protein count of 15 grams, and a total of 542.6 calories (full vitamin, mineral, and enzyme packed calories).

Remember that heat causes irreversible changes in protein that downgrade the protein, making it less nutritious. This is one reason why we recommend uncooked food.

¼ avocado
7 slices of cucumber
1 cup of mung sprouts
½ cup summer squash
2 T. sunflower seeds

½ cup leafy greens
1/8 cup salad oil
2 slices tomato or red
  pepper
Small bits of dulse or kelp

Use the salad oil in making the "herb dressing" (below) and toss. You may eat any one of the items or more, untossed.

HERB DRESSING

¼ tsp. thyme (ground)
¼ tsp. marjoram
  (ground)
¼ tsp. tarragon (ground)
½ tsp. basil (ground)

½ cup cold pressed oil
3 T. apple cider vinegar
1 T. finely chopped fresh
  parsley
½ tsp. sea salt (or 1 tsp.
  kelp)

Shake vigorously in covered jar till blended. Allow to stand in refrigerator till flavors are blended.

Garnishes add to the salad's interest. For vegetable or main-dish salads, use pimiento, green or red pepper strips, radishes, watercress, parsley or mint sprigs, carrot or celery curls, twisted lemon slices, chives or other fresh herbs.

GARLIC HERB DRESSING

Use the same basic recipe as in the Lemon Herb Dressing, eliminating the lemon juice, add ⅔ cup apple cider vinegar, ¼ tsp. dry mustard, and 1 clove garlic, peeled and split. After the flavors are blended, the garlic may be discarded (a day or two later).

PICKIN' SALAD WITH GUACAMOLE DIP

celery sticks	radishes
carrot sticks	sliced turnips
zucchini sticks	sliced beets
cherry tomatoes	raw broccoli slices

On a large round platter, arrange in eight sections around the outside of the platter. Set dish of guacamole dip in the center.

GUACAMOLE DIP

2 or 3 ripe avocadoes
1 tomato chopped
   and mashed
1T. kelp

½ onion chopped fine
hot peppers chopped fine
2 tsp. vegetable seasoning

Mash avocadoes, stir in rest of ingredients to taste. This may be thinned a little with Rejuvelac to make a salad dressing.

THE LIQUID SALAD

¾ cup finely chopped
   onion
¾ tsp. minced garlic
1½ cup bell pepper,
   finely chopped
3½ cups fresh tomatoes
   diced

1 T. paprika
1 T. olive oil
½ cup fresh lemon juice
1 cup water
½ cup thinly sliced
   cucumbers
1 T. kelp

Blend and chill 2-3 hrs. Add cucumber just before serving.

POTATO AND CARROT SALAD

1 carrot grated
1 medium unpeeled potato
   shredded
1 tsp. chopped onion

1 tsp. olive oil
½ mashed avocado
minced parsley, cayenne,
   and paprika to taste

Mix all ingredients together. Serve in a lettuce cup. Sprinkle with dill seed, sunflower seeds or sesame seeds.

GADO GADO—INDONESIAN VEGETABLE SALAD

3 peeled carrots, cut in matchsticks
½ lb. fresh young green beans, cut in thin diagonals

4 cups shredded salad greens (lettuce, escarole, kale, spinach)
1 lb. fresh bean sprouts
1 tomato cut in wedges
3 medium potatoes, diced

Arrange greens on a large platter. Arrange carrots, potatoes, green beans, and bean sprouts in rows on greens. Garnish with tomatoes. Serve with Sesame Seed sauce.

STUFFED PEPPER

1 sweet bell pepper, halved and seeded
red and green cabbage sliced thin
tomato cut in small pieces

celery chopped
dill to season
lecinaise (bought at Health Food Store)

Mix sliced cabbage, tomato, celery, and dill. Add enough lecinaise to moisten. Pile cabbage slaw inside halves of pepper.

CAULIFLOWER PEPPER

raw cauliflowerets sliced
chopped bell peppers

watercress or parsley
soya-lecithin mayonnaise
(bought at Health Food
Store)

Mix all ingredients with Soya-lecithin mayonnaise and serve on a bed of greens.

DELUXE SPROUT SALAD

1 cup of your favorite
   sprouts
½ cup grated celery
½ cup diced onions
½ cup grated carrots

1 diced red pepper
leaf lettuce
avocado
tomato
lemon juice
kelp
vegetable seasoning

Combine the sprouts, celery, onions, carrots and red pepper. Mix thoroughly in a large bowl. Toss with fresh lemon juice, kelp and vegetable seasoning. Serve on leaf lettuce and garnish with avocado and tomato.

GREEK SALAD SUPPER

2 medium potatoes
1 T. each minced parsley
and green onion
1 T. salad oil (cold pressed)
½ T. apple cider vinegar,
kelp and vegetable sea-
soning
1/6 cup lecinaise
¼ red onion, separated in
rings (thinly sliced)

¼ bunch watercress,
rinsed, drained, chopped
2 cups shredded salad
greens (escarole, chicory
and lettuce)
1 large tomato, cut in wedges
½ avocado sliced
½ cucumber cut in spears
½ bell pepper, seeded,
sliced in rings
½ bunch radishes, cleaned

Slice potatoes, toss with parsley, green onion, oil, vinegar, kelp and vegetable seasoning; add lecinaise. Chill until ready to serve. Arrange bed of watercress and greens on platter. Mound potatoes in center and arrange tomato wedges, avocado, cucumber, bell pepper and onion on greens surrounding potato salad. Have a side dish of sunflower seeds and pumpkin seeds. Have Herb Dressing available.

CUCUMBER SALAD DRESSING

1 cup lecinaise
pinch of dill

½ cup cucumber

Blend in blender until smooth. Good on tossed salad.

GREEN SALAD DRESSING

2 cups spinach (or indoor greens from sprouts growing one week in light)
1 cup of water
½ avocado

4 T. sunflower seed meal (finely ground sunflower seeds)
1 T. kelp
Vegetable seasoning to taste

Put water in blender, drop in other ingredients, blending to desired consistency.

SAUERKRAUT
(A fermented food rich in enzymes)

cabbage, red or green or both

Thyme, dill, kelp

For variety, juniper berries, carrots, peppers, onions or beets can be added.

Cut vegetables in strips or grate. Layer cabbage in the bottom of a large earthenware pot or crock about 6 inches deep, then sprinkle a handful of juniper berries, then a layer of carrots, a layer of peppers, beets, and onions, then layer of cabbage, etc. Just cabbage can be done alone if you prefer.

Each layer should be pressed down so that the cabbage will be saturated in its own juice. Repeat the procedure. When the container is full, cover with a clean cloth and a heavy stone cover or a cloth, plate and weight.

About once a week, remove the cloth, wash and

replace it. Keep the pot in the kitchen at room temperature for about three weeks (or in a cellar or other storage place). Then remove the foam or mildew from the top; the sauerkraut is ready to eat. Store it in glass jars in the refrigerator. Start your next sauerkraut again in the empty pot. You will improve the making of it if you keep it up.

Some people like one week old sauerkraut. Taste for yourself.

HUNZA BREAD
For special occasions or guests only

5 parts whole wheat flour   1 part barley
1 part rye   1 part buckwheat groats
1 part oats   1 part millet

Grind the seeds to flour if necessary. Mix all ingredients well. Add enough water to make a medium dough. Take a ball of dough about the size of an orange and flatten in hands to 5'' diameter and ¾'' thick. Prick with fork. (Important to keep it from exploding in the oven) and bake at 350 degrees for 30-40 minutes.

WHEAT GUM, CEREAL & MILK

Take one day wheat sprouts, a handful, and chew until it is the consistency of gum...a delightful, healthy gum.
—The soaked wheat that is used to make Rejuvelac, kept without water for 15 hours will sprout slightly and may be used to make a breakfast cereal, a milk, gum, or plant to produce wheatgrass.
—Use soaked wheat around plants for fertilizer or worm food.
—To make the delicious cereal, blend one cup of the slightly sprouted wheat seeds and ½ to 1 cup of water until the consistency you enjoy.
—To make the tasty milk, blend together one cup of the slightly sprouted wheat and two cups of warm water and strain.

HUNZA PIZZA

Use Hunza bread recipe and roll very thin to fit round pizza pan. Bake in 350 degree oven for 20 minutes. Spread with red salsa taco sauce. Sprinkle with chopped bell peppers, chopped tomatoes, chopped hot peppers, chopped celery, onions, squash, avocado, garlic and/or broccoli, mushrooms, and egg plant (all raw).

9 | COMTEMPLATIONS

In our present day, for the majority of the people who turn up with malignant cancer, it is synonymous in meaning with "terminal disease," a matter of waiting to die. In relating my experiences in this book, it is my hope that some other person in reading it will be helped to survive the nightmare of cancer, and be shown a way to live instead.

Although it is a lot easier to say now than when I was going through it, a lot of good has come out of my having had cancer. One major thing, of course, was the regaining of my health through the wheatgrass therapy and the "living foods" diet. But even more than this, I am grateful for my being faced with the reality of death. I had to prepare for it. I was forced to do some real soul-searching and found something missing. I came up with many questions, but no answers! My finding the answers to these questions was the most exciting and rewarding thing of all, so I want to share with you, in capsule form, some of the meaning that has come into my life as a consequence.

The average person just never gets around to thinking about his own death. I don't mean morbid, fearful, contemplation of death, but really coming to grips with the question, "What is death?" which inevitably leads to the question, "What is life?" Anthropologists, philosophers, historians, scholars in every walk of life have written books, poems and treatises on these profound mysteries for many centuries now, and have not come up with very satisfactory answers.

Knowledge is highly exalted in the world today. Educational institutions are mass producing "educated" people. But am I really educated if I don't know what life is, why I am alive, where I am going, what death is, whether death is the end of it all or whether there is really something beyond death?

These questions began to haunt me when I came face to face with the very real possibility that the last curtain was coming down on my life. Due to circumstances which I believe to be beyond coincidence, I now believe that man can know, and I have found some answers and am in the process of finding more.

Religion did not play an important part in my early life. As a child I attended Sunday School when I felt like it.

At the age of thirteen, I was orphaned. This brought about my living in a home where everyone attended Sunday School and church regularly, so I did as was expected of me.

Arn was brought up in a religious home and attended Sunday School and church regularly.

We met in church at the age of fifteen. As young people, we had both accepted Jesus Christ as our saviour and believed that the Christian life was the way for us. We married at age nineteen.

At nineteen, we had not yet accepted the fact that Christians were imperfect. This raised many disturbing, unanswered questions, especially when we looked at other so-called Christians and the church leaders, evangelists, etc. and could see the many flaws. Weren't Christians supposed to be patterning their lives after Christ and as a consequence, living the way a person should live? Weren't ministers of the gospel supposed to have a large enough vision to encompass believers everywhere, in other churches as well as his own denomination's missionaries, and other people who love Jesus Christ without splitting doctrinal hairs? We thought so, but we didn't find it.

We hadn't yet learned, as we are able to see today, that every believer is in a different stage of spiritual growth, including the ministers as well as the doubting Thomases. Being rather observant, analytical and perhaps critical, early in our marriage we became discouraged by our doubts and questions arising from what appeared to us to be hypocrisy all around us in the church. It wasn't too long before we took the easy way out and decided church was not for us.

We became very self-reliant, with much confidence in our own abilities. You might say that "logic" became our god. Arn made the statement many times that he felt that logic was the only method of intelligently determining destiny. We didn't object to religion or churches being in the world, or a part of other people's lives (like Arn's family). It was just that we didn't need it. I've heard Arn say that he didn't think the masses could control themselves without religion to keep them in line. It would be an impossible world to live in if their churches were not their consciences. Our children were not raised in the church. You might even say that we became agnostics. Years passed.

Then when I developed cancer, I was faced with death, and I wasn't ready to die. When I thought about it, I realized that the only certain factor about life is that sooner or later it will end in death.

Perhaps the first little ray of light that began dawning on me started in Boston at the "mansion." I went to Boston with an open mind seeking some answers which my self-sufficiency had failed to bring to me. I had become well aware of the fact that I didn't have the answer that was going to enable me to live, nor did I have the answer or answers that would enable me to face death in peace—so I was searching.

Ann Wigmore is a very religious person and is always planting seeds. Not only organic ones to be sprouted, or to make wheatgrass, but in an attempt to stretch a person's mind to include God in every aspect of living. She always gave thanks to God before eating any meal because she is truly thankful, not only for daily "manna" but for all that she believes God has shown her in her work, and for the miracles of good health that her work in turn has brought to many. She has incorporated religious books in her library at the mansion right next to the books on nutrition, available to all who come there.

We explored the books on nutrition, but left the others alone. We were used to having grace said at Arn's family's homes, so we had no problem being politely accommodating in that area, but due to our former rejection of religion, we were really not open to the possibility that any of these ideas were a part of our answer.

However, the ray of hope for my return to health that began in Boston, especially having come about through such a natural method, began to stretch our minds in more ways than one.

Perhaps, in our self-sufficiency we had closed our minds to other areas of life that needed opening. I know so well our impatience with the many physicians who seem to have closed their minds to any treatment of cancer other than surgery, radiation, and chemotherapy. Maybe there were other things we had been missing because of prematurely closing our minds. These thoughts were in the back of my mind one Sunday morning as we were eating breakfast.

For years, a vital interest in Arn's life has been the study of world and national economics. He has had a long standing concern for what is happening to our economy, and has studied many books on the subject, as well as experiencing the economic ups and downs of leading a very active business life. He has personally felt the heavy hand of government bureaucracy and the almost unchecked power of the labor unions at work in the business world. Because of this, he has become somewhat of a business and economic expert, with amazing accuracy in his predictions. Arn has regularly formulated and predicted the coming events of monetary crises, depression, civil insurrections, etc. simply from the history of the facts and his knowledge of the present trends. Imagine our surprise when Arn turned on the television (something we never did on a Sunday morning) and there was an evangelist making all the same predictions that Arn had been making, but for entirely different reasons.

I guess it's human nature that most everyone likes to have someone else agree with them in the way that they think, but an evangelist? Aren't they supposed to be busy thinking about saving souls and interpreting scriptures? Here was an evangelist coming up with the same conclusions, based on his twenty-seven years of studying prophecy from the Bible, that Arn had determined on his own. How could studying prophecy from the scriptures tell us what was happening today? Incredible. Too hard to believe, but naturally this sparked our interest and we listened.

As we listened, we heard him teach many things that we already knew from Arn's studying, things like:

"There are two opposing forces vying for the domination of the world in existence today. One is the world of freedom-loving, free enterprisers, who teach all men should be able to decide their own financial and circumstantial fate. The other is the dictatorship of

Communism that teaches that the supreme control of man and his circumstances should be left with government and that the government should decide who does what and what each owns and possesses."

Then he went on to explain:

"No one doubts any more that there will be another World War. We only ask in our hearts, when, who, why, and what will be the outcome? The Bible is very clear as to who will be involved in the next World War. The Scriptures also clearly indicate who will win and why they will be fighting so intensely (Ezekiel 38 and 39). God has chosen in His infinite wisdom to reveal to His sons and daughters of the last period of time, prior to these devastating events, these facts concerning what is coming. He has declared what would happen and told us to prepare ourselves for it. He also tells how to prepare for this world shattering, global catastrophe of war."

His knowledge of the ancient historical names of the countries involved in the drama of the Middle East, Europe and Asia suddenly brought the prophecies of Ezekiel 38 and 39 alive, and added a new dimension to our thinking.

Consequently, we began to tune into his program regularly. Then one evening we took the opportunity to spend a few hours listening to this evangelist in person. Our real interest was in his theories on the dollar devaluations and on the role of gold and silver in the coming economic chaos. However, he brought the Bible alive in other areas, also, and began to interest us in many facets of things to come. We found our old reservations and former stumbling blocks dropping away. Before the evening was over, he asked for hands to be raised by those who were ready to meet their Lord at His coming for them. Many hands flew up with enthusiasm, but not ours. We simply could not commit ourselves without further study.

Arn and I have heard many politicians predicting optimistic solutions to our country's problems, other politicians predicting nothing but disaster. We've heard scientists predict that the world will be so overpopulated in another ten years that a major part of us will die of starvation. Then we've heard geologists predict we are running out of minerals in the earth that are vitally needed to keep civilization going and that when we do, we are all doomed. We've heard others say Communism will completely rule the world in ten years time. How does a person know whom to believe?

Based on logic, Arn's original economic predictions foresaw what is happening, but he could find *no solutions* to the continual decay of our freedoms, of our monetary system, and of our government. According to his thinking, there wasn't time to re-educate the people, there was no way to stop the collision course that we are on. He could predict the disastrous outcome that is coming, but could not see the opportunity for rebuilding what some authors seem to believe will eventually happen. Arn could see no way for a happy ending.

When our interest was provoked by what this evangelist had had to say, we decided to see for ourselves if this ancient manuscript, the Bible, really had anything to say about the present day in which we live.

Both having analytical minds, we decided to make a detailed study of prophecy first. Again, we piled into research materials as if our lives depended on it. For the first time, we took time to really look into the Bible with an open mind and studied it for ourselves. I don't think that we have ever studied anything together that is more interesting or enlightening. We have tried to be honest with ourselves and as objective as possible. When we came across something that did not seem to make sense, we set it aside as something to study deeper at a later date, rather than throw out the whole Bible because our understanding only went so far at that time. (These deeper study areas are gradually clearing up, one by one). Our research has shown us to our satisfaction that biblical prophecies were just as accurate in the past as it appeared they would be in the future. We could trace some of them happening right then, (and now) and it was with utter amazement that we watched the puzzle pieces coming together. After discovering this, we found it easy to believe all the words in the Bible. We have tried hard not to be caught up in something simply for the sake of finding answers. It has been very exciting and at times mind boggling.

In the past, we had placed the hard-core Bible believers in the realm of the dreamers, or fairy-tale believers, or deluded extremists, but concentrated study has us seeing the tremendous foundation of history that walks hand in glove with the Old and the New Testaments. We found our faith being restored by trying to be as open-minded as possible to the questions in our minds instead of carelessly assuming that the Bible teaches hundreds of conflicting ideas. It has been a real challenge to sort them out and dig for real truth and meaning.

After really wrestling with our studies, our minds, and our prejudices, many of our former doubts and disillusionments have been cleared up in regard to Christianity and the body of believers. Contentions by many of the denominations that you had to belong to their church in order to get to "heaven" had been one of our major hang-ups. We couldn't see a just God engineering that kind of a system.

Our study has caused Arn and me to give up our hostility towards God and His Word. We now believe that a wise and merciful God *has* caused the Bible (we believe the Bible to be the book of truth) to be written and that all one needs to do is to see and believe the truth (sometimes after a long search) and he will share in the glorious plans of the future.

Many months after our studies began, we again availed ourselves of the opportunity to listen to this evangelist teach in person. This time when he asked for a show of hands, happily we could raise ours.

We have come to believe that the important thing is our personal relationship with God, not to which church a person belongs. We have surrendered our lives to Him.

I am no longer afraid to die. My questions about the future have been answered to my satisfaction, and it's the most fascinating adventure I have ever experienced just watching it all unfold. Life has a new meaning and a happiness never before known.

Too much has happened starting with my cancer, all in sequence, to be a coincidence. Have you ever heard the story of the mule? First you hit him over the head to get his attention. Well, I believe that God allowed (not caused) me to go through all this to get my attention. When I finally gave in, I could see the plan. He led me through all of our logical solutions to my breast cancer, none of which worked. In my darkest hour, out of the blue, He led me to Boston, on the whisper of a chance, a crazy far-out idea that "wheatgrass" and "living foods" could be my answer to defeating cancer, which unbelievably proved to be true. I believe God led us to watch the television program that sparked our interest in studying prophecy which in turn led us to becoming His children again after having turned our backs on Him for so many years. What joy to have the inner peace that only God can give!

We have come to see that it is not a matter of patterning our lives after Christ at all, but of having the power of Christ within us to lead the kind of lives God would have us lead *when we yield to that power*. Even as Christians we still have to choose each day whether we are going to live up to the light within us.

When I think now of how we thought the Christian life was for the weak and for the dreamers, I can really laugh at us. No way. One thing for sure, the Christian life is not the easy way out. There's no room for stubborn pride, nor fear, nor for looking at where the next person has fallen down, but when we remember to keep looking to God in Jesus Christ, it's uphill again, and is indeed the greatest adventure of all in our lives.

My last "hold out" came at an unexpected time. I had carried a bitter resentment for a couple of years, and one afternoon while studying the Bible, out of the blue it came, "I know that I can forgive them!" Immediately, it was like a tremendous burden was lifted from me, and I was set free!

The freedom of which I speak can not be decreed by a government. Government can put me in physical and economic slavery and I would still have this freedom. It is a freedom of the spirit. Jesus Christ has set me free, and no man, or government can ever take that from me.

APPENDIX

FOOTNOTES

CHAPTER TWO
1. *Time*, March 19, 1973

CHAPTER THREE
1. F. E., Adair, Role of Surgery and Irradiation in Cancer of Breast, J.A.M.A. 121:553, 1943
2. G. Keynes, (Quoting a discussion of Murley, R.S.) Proc. Cardiff M. Soc., P. 40, 1954.
3. Virginia Wuerthele-Caspe Livingston, M.D., *Cancer: A New Breakthrough*, Los Angeles, Nash Publishing Corp.

CHAPTER FIVE
1. *Encyclopedia of Organic Gardening*, Rodale Books, Inc., Emmaus, Penna. 18049.
2. Ibid.
3. Ibid.
4. Ann Wigmore, D.D.,N.D., *Be Your Own Doctor —Let Living Foods Be Your Medicine.*

CHAPTER SEVEN
1. Ann Wigmore, D.D.N.D., *Be Your Own Doctor— Let Living Foods Be Your Medicine.*
2. Ann Wigmore, D.D., *Garden Indoors.*
3. *Science News Letter*, May 22, 1943.
4. Catharyn Elwood, *Feel Like a Million.*

RECOMMENDED READING AND REFERENCES

The following are books that you may find useful.

Balch, James F.; Balch, Phyllis A., *Prescription for Nutritional Healing*. Avery Publishing Group., Garden City Park, New York, 1990.

Blauer, Stephen. *The Juicing Book.* Avery Publishing Group., Garden City Park, New York, 1985.

Calbom, Cherie; Keane, Maureen. *Juicing for Life.* Avery Publishing Group., Garden City Park, New York, 1992.

Fink, John M. Fink., *Third Opinion: An International Directory to Alternative Therapy Centers for the Treatment and Prevention of Cancer and Other Degenerative Diseases.* Avery Publishing Group., Garden City Park, New York, 1992.

Howell, Edward., *Enzyme Nutrition.* Avery Publishing Group., Garden City Park, New York, 1985.

Jensen, Bernard. *Foods That Heal.* Avery Publishing Group., Garden City Park, New York, 1988.

Kendall, Francis. *Sweet Temptation Natural Dessert Book.* Avery Publishing Group., Garden City Park, New York, 1986.

Lieberman, Shari; Bruning, Nancy. *The Real Vitamin and Mineral Book.* Avery Publishing Group., Garden City Park, New York, 1990.

Walker, N.W., *Raw Vegetable Juices.* Norwalk Press., Phoenix, Arizona.1971

Wigmore, Ann. *Be Your Own Doctor.* Avery Publishing Group., Garden City Park, New York, 1982.

Wigmore, Ann. *Hippocrates Diet and Health Program.* Avery Publishing Group., Garden City Park, New York, 1984.

Wigmore, Ann. *Recipes For Longer Life.* Avery Publishing Group., Garden City Park, New York, 1978.

Wigmore, Ann. *The Healing Power Within.* Avery Publishing Group., Garden City Park, New York, 1985.

Wigmore, Ann. *Hippocrates Diet and Health Program.* Avery Publishing Group., Garden City Park, New York, 1984.

Wigmore, Ann. *The Sprouting Book.* Avery Publishing Group., Garden City Park, New York, 1986.

Wigmore, Ann. *The Wheat Grass Book.* Avery Publishing Group., Garden City Park, New York, 1985.

Wigmore, Ann. *Why Suffer?* Avery Publishing Group., Garden City Park, New York, 1985.

To learn more about the Living Food Program you can contact the following organizations:

Ann Wigmore Foundation
196 Commonwealth Avenue
Boston, MA 02116
(617) 267-9424

Ann Wigmore Institute
P.O. Box 429
Rincon, PR 00677
(809) 868-6307

Hippocrates Health Institute
1443 Palmdale Court
West Palm Beach, FL 33411
(407) 471-8876

Creative Health Institute
918 Union City Road
Union City, MI 49094
(517) 278-6260

Optimum Health Institute
of San Diego
6970 Central Avenue
Lemon Grove, CA 91945
(619) 464-3346

INDEX